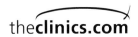

CRITICAL CARE NURSING CLINICS OF NORTH AMERICA

Cardiovascular Disease in Women

GUEST EDITOR
Lynn Smith Schnautz, RN, MSN,
CCRN, CCNS, NP-C

DISCARD

CONSULTING EDITOR
Janet Foster, PhD, RN, CNS, CCRN

September 2008 • Volume 20 • Number 3

SAUNDERS

An Imprint of Elsevier, Inc.
PHILADELPHIA   LONDON   TORONTO   MONTREAL   SYDNEY   TOKYO

W.B. SAUNDERS COMPANY
A Division of Elsevier Inc.

Elsevier Inc., 1600 John F. Kennedy Blvd., Suite 1800, Philadelphia, PA 19103-2899.

http://www.theclinics.com

CRITICAL CARE NURSING CLINICS OF NORTH AMERICA
September 2008
Editor: Ali Gavenda

Volume 20, Number 3
ISSN 0899-5885
ISBN-13: 978-1-4160-6283-7
ISBN-10: 1-4160-6283-1

Critical Care Nursing Clinics of North America (ISSN 0899-5885) is published quarterly by Elsevier Inc., 360 Park Avenue South, New York, NY 10010-1710. Months of issue are March, June, September, and December. Business and Editorial Offices: 1600 John F. Kennedy Blvd., Suite 1800, Philadelphia, PA 19103-2899. Customer Service Office: 6277 Sea Harbor Drive, Orlando, FL 32887-4800. Periodicals postage paid at New York, NY and additional mailing offices. Subscription prices are $120.00 per year for US individuals, $212.00 per year for US institutions, $63.00 per year for US students and residents, $155.00 per year for Canadian individuals, $260.00 per year for Canadian institutions, $166.00 per year for international individuals, $260.00 per year for international institutions and $86.00 per year for Canadian and foreign students/residents. To receive student/resident rate, orders must be accompanied by name of affiliated institution, data of term, and the *signature* of program/residency coordinator on institution letterhead. Orders will be billed at individual rate until proof of status is received. Foreign air speed delivery is included in all *Clinics* subscription prices. All prices are subject to change without notice. **POSTMASTER:** Send address changes to *Critical Care Nursing Clinics of North America*, Elsevier Periodicals Customer Service, 6277 Sea Harbor Drive, Orlando, FL 32887-4800. **Customer Service: 1-800-654-2452 (US). From outside of the US, call 1-407-563-6020. Fax: 1-407-363-9661. E-mail: JournalsCustomerService-usa@elsevier.com.**

Reprints. For copies of 100 or more of articles in this publication, please contact the Commercial Reprints Department, Elsevier Inc., 360 Park Avenue South, New York, New York, 10010-1710; Tel.: (212) 633-3813, Fax: (212) 462-1935, and E-mail: reprints@elsevier.com.

Critical Care Nursing Clinics of North America is covered in *MEDLINE/PubMed (Index Medicus), International Nursing Index, Nursing Citation Index, Cumulative Index to Nursing and Allied Health Literature,* and *RNdex Top 100.*

Printed in the United States of America.

CONSULTING EDITOR

JANET FOSTER, PhD, RN, CNS, CCRN, Assistant Professor, College of Nursing, Texas Woman's University, Houston, Texas

GUEST EDITOR

LYNN SMITH SCHNAUTZ, RN, MSN, CCRN, CCNS, NP-C, Cardiovascular Clinical Nurse Specialist, Deaconess Hospital; and Family Nurse Practitioner, Integrity Family Physicians, Evansville, Indiana

CONTRIBUTORS

LORI BARRON, BSN, RN, BC, Team Leader, Cardiac Rehabilitation, Deaconess Hospital, Evansville, Indiana

JERRY BECKER, MD, FACCP, Cardiologist; and Medical Director, Lipid Clinic, The Heart Group, Evansville, Indiana

JANET BRUNETTI, RN, CNRN, Deaconess Hopsital, Evansville, Indiana

DAMON B. COTTRELL, MS, RN, CCNS, CCRN, CNS-BC, CEN, Clinical Nurse Specialist, Cardiology, Washington Hospital Center, Washington, District of Columbia

KELLI S. DEMPSEY, MSN, APRN-BC, AOCNP, Oncology Nurse Practitioner, American Cancercare, Evansville, Indiana

MISSIE ELPERS, MS, Lipid Clinic Manager, The Heart Group, Evansville, Indiana

CHERYL HERRMANN, RN, MS, APN, CCRN, CCNS-CSC/CMC, Cardiac Clinical Nurse Specialist, Methodist Medical Center of Illinois, Peoria, Illinois

ROBERTA E. HOEBEKE, RN, PhD, FNP-BC, Associate Professor of Nursing, College of Nursing and Health Professions, University of Southern Indiana, Evansville, Indiana

MICHELLE M. JONES, MSN, RN, ACNP-BC, ANP, Nurse Practitioner, Interventional Radiology, Georgetown University Medical Center, Washington, District of Columbia

BERYL KEEGAN, RN, MSN/Ed, CCRN, CLNC, Professor, Department of Nursing, Medical Careers Institute, School of Health Science, ECPI College of Technology, Newport News, Virginia

PATRICIA LEGGETT, RN, BSN, CCRN, CMSRN, Clinical Nurse IV, Deaconess Hospital, Evansville, Indiana

ANGELA L. PRUITT, MSN, RN, CNS, Clinical Nurse Specialist, Cardiovascular Renal Care Center, Deaconess Hospital, Evansville, Indiana

DAWN ROWLEY, RN, Clinical Nurse IV, Deaconess Hospital, Evansville, Indiana

LYNN SMITH SCHNAUTZ, RN, MSN, CCRN, CCNS, NP-C, Cardiovascular Clinical Nurse Specialist, Deaconess Hospital; and Family Nurse Practitioner, Integrity Family Physicians, Evansville, Indiana

MARY JANE SWARTZ, RN, MSN, ACNS-BC, Adjunct Faculty, University of Southern Indiana, Evansville, Indiana; and Adjunct Faculty, Henderson Community College, Henderson, Kentucky

EUGENIA WELCH, BSN, RN, CCRN, Staff Nurse, Emergency Department, Presbyterian Hospital of Kaufman, Kaufman, Texas

CONTENTS

The American Hospital Association's Guidelines for Cardiopulmonary Resuscitation and Emergency Cardiovascular Care 2005 were announced in November 2005. One of the most significant changes in the 2005 guidelines was the simplification of cardiopulmonary resuscitation instruction, which emphasizes reducing the frequency and length of interruption of chest compressions and increasing the number of compressions delivered per minute. This article outlines the guidelines' recommendations with particular attention to defibrillation, cardiac arrest, and symptomatic bradycardia and tachycardia.

Even though a woman has a one in two lifetime risk of dying from a coronary event, women and health care providers do not realize that heart disease is the greatest health risk for women. The purpose of this article is to increase awareness of women and heart disease. The article summarizes the evidence-based literature regarding the epidemiology of heart disease in women, risk factors and risk factor stratification, symptoms, diagnosis, and treatment. The text includes the American Heart Association's 2007 Evidenced Based Guidelines for Cardiovascular Disease Prevention.

Kawasaki disease is the leading cause of acquired heart disease in children. Little is known about the origin; however, speculation exists that the disease is associated with the use of carpet cleaner or stagnate water. The disease can have devastating lifelong effects on the heart and cardiovascular system. Early recognition of the clinical manifestations by the health care provider may lead to early treatment and prevention of long-term cardiovascular disease. This article presents a case study, with discussion about the prevalence, incidence, pathophysiology, clinical features, and collaborative clinical management of Kawasaki disease.

differences in risk factors for these dysrhythmias will help guide treatment decisions. As new knowledge is gained through research, practitioners can provide gender-specific care to women who have or are at increased risk of cardiac dysrhythmia.

particularly by women and the elderly. The goals of CR are to improve the physiologic and psychosocial condition of the patient. Understanding the benefits of an effective CR program will help critical care nurses and physicians promote and refer patients who have cardiovascular disease to this life-changing heart healthy program. This article identifies the components and benefits of a successful CR program.

FORTHCOMING ISSUES

RECENT ISSUES

ELSEVIER
SAUNDERS

Crit Care Nurs Clin N Am 20 (2008) xi–xii

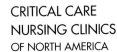
CRITICAL CARE
NURSING CLINICS
OF NORTH AMERICA

Preface

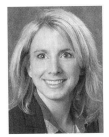

Lynn Smith Schnautz, RN, MSN, CCRN, CCNS, NP-C
Guest Editor

Heart disease is the leading cause of death in the United States, killing almost 700,000 Americans each year. Nearly 500,000 of those deaths are attributed to coronary artery disease. Women are at risk for heart disease and heart attacks, just like men. In fact, heart disease is the leading cause of death among women over 65 years of age. American women are four to six times more likely to die of heart disease than of breast cancer, and heart disease kills more women over 65 years of age than all cancers combined [1]. In addition to being the major cause of death in women, heart disease may lead to a significantly decreased quality of life. Heart attacks in the postmenopausal years and cardiomyopathies and valvular heart disease in the premenopausal years carry serious health consequences for women that may affect their quality of life. Some forms of heart disease may be more difficult to recognize and treat in women than in men [2].

The important topic of heart disease in women has received inadequate attention from patients, physicians, advanced practice nurses, other health care providers and the community in general during the past two decades. Two national programs, however, have been launched to increase women's awareness about the number one killer of women. In 2003 the First Lady, Laura Bush, introduced "The Heart Truth" and served as a Heart Truth Ambassador, helping lead the crusade to educate women regarding heart disease. At Fashion Week 2003, the "Red Dress" was introduced as the national symbol for awareness of heart disease in women [3]. In February 2004, the American Heart Association's "Go Red for Women, Love Your Heart" national movement began to educate the public and healthcare professionals about the number one killer of women and the prevention tactics that should be used to prevent heart disease in women [4].

This issue of *Critical Care Nursing Clinics of North America* is devoted to heart disease in women. Early prevention and recognition are the keys to optimizing outcomes. It introduces women wearing many different styles of "Red Dresses," with the hope that you will recognize her when she presents to your clinical practice.

I thank all of the contributors for sharing their time, talents, and expertise regarding heart

disease in women. I hope that all women who
have heart disease will be diagnosed and treated
early, at the first signs of heart disease. I wish
you well as you read these pages, acquire
knowledge, and incorporate this evidence into
your clinical practice.

Lynn Smith Schnautz, RN, MSN, CCRN,
CCNS, NP-C
Cardiovascular Clinical Nurse Specialist
Deaconess Hospital
600 Mary Street
Evansville, IN 47747, USA

and

Family Nurse Practitioner
Integrity Family Physicians
6221 East Physicians Court
Evansville, IN 47715, USA

E-mail address: lynn_schnautz@deaconess.com

References

[1] U.S. Department of Health and Human Services Office on Women's Health. Heart Disease 2007. Available at: http://womenshealth.gov/faq/heartdis.htm. Accessed November 14, 2007.
[2] Wilansky S, Willerson JT. Heart disease in women. Philadelphia: Churchill Livingstone; 2002.
[3] The Heart Truth Web site. Available at: http://www.nhlbi.nih.gov/health/hearttruth/. Accessed January 30, 2008.
[4] American Heart Association Go For Red Web site. Available at: www.goredforwomen.org. Accessed January 30, 2008.

ELSEVIER
SAUNDERS

CRITICAL CARE
NURSING CLINICS
OF NORTH AMERICA

Crit Care Nurs Clin N Am 20 (2008) 245–250

A Brief Overview of Some of the Changes of the American Heart Association's Guidelines for Cardiopulmonary Resuscitation and Emergency Cardiovascular Care

Janet Brunetti, RN, CNRN

Deaconess Hospital, 600 Mary Street, Evansville, IN 47747, USA

Many women believe that heart disease is something that happens to someone else. The following facts regarding women and cardiovascular disease can be found on the American Heart Association's (AHA) Web site [1]:

- "Cardiovascular disease (CVD) ranks first among all disease categories in hospital discharges for women.
- Nearly 39 percent of all female deaths in America occur from CVD, which includes coronary heart disease (CHD), stroke, and other cardiovascular diseases.
- CVD is a particularly important problem among minority women. The death rate due to CVD is substantially higher in black women than in white women.
- In 2003, CVD claimed the lives of 483,842 females; cancer (all forms combined) 267,902.
- In 2003, coronary heart disease claimed the lives of 233,886 females, compared with 41,566 lives from breast cancer and 67,894 from lung cancer.
- 38 percent of women die within one year after a heart attack.
- Stroke is a leading cause of serious, long-term disability; an estimated 15 to 30 percent of stroke survivors are permanently disabled.
- Misperceptions still exist that CVD is not a real problem for women."

The Centers for Disease Control's Web site shares the following facts [2]:

- In the United States one woman in four dies from heart disease, whereas 1 in 30 dies from breast cancer.
- "Twenty-three percent of women die within 1 year after having a heart attack.
- Within 6 years of having a heart attack, about 46% of women become disabled with heart failure.
- Two thirds of women who have a heart attack fail to make a full recovery."

Awareness and prevention are important, but what should one do when someone suffers a heart attack or brain attack (stroke)? According to the 2005 AHA 2005 Guidelines for Cardiopulmonary Resuscitation and Emergency Cardiovascular Care, "Sudden cardiac arrest is a leading cause of death in the United States and Canada" [3]. Responding quickly with evidenced-based interventions can make the difference between life and death. Following is a brief overview of some of the changes in the AHA 2005 guidelines, which can be found on line at www.circulationaha.org.

The AHA's Guidelines for Cardiopulmonary Resuscitation and Emergency Cardiovascular Care 2005 were announced in November 2005. The 2005 guidelines "are based on the evidence evaluation from the 2005 International Consensus Conference on Cardiopulmonary Resuscitation and Emergency Cardiovascular Care Science with Treatment Recommendations, hosted by the American Heart Association in Dallas, Texas,

E-mail address: janet_brunetti@deaconess.com

0899-5885/08/$ - see front matter © 2008 Elsevier Inc. All rights reserved.
doi:10.1016/j.ccell.2008.03.009

January 23–30, 2005" [4]. The guidelines "are based on the most extensive review of CPR [cardiopulmonary resuscitation] yet published" [4]. The 2005 guidelines "have been streamlined to reduce the amount of information that rescuers need to learn and remember to clarify the most important skills that rescuers need to perform" [4]. The International Liaison Committee on Resuscitation (ILCOR) collaborated to develop an evidence-based consensus to guide worldwide resuscitation practices and to review resuscitation science. The ILCOR is "an international consortium of representatives from many of the world's resuscitation councils" [4]. After the 2005 Consensus Conference, AHA experts on emergency cardiovascular care "adapted the ILCOR scientific statements and expanded the treatment recommendations to construct these new guidelines" [4].

Changes in cardiopulmonary resuscitation

One of the most significant changes in the 2005 guidelines was the simplification of CPR instruction, which emphasizes reducing the frequency and length of interruption of chest compressions and increasing the number of compressions delivered per minute. Interruption in chest compressions should be minimized, and the rate of compressions in infants, children, and adults should be about 100 per minute. The steps of CPR for lay rescuers were simplified so that the steps of CPR for the adult, child, and infant victims are more similar and therefore are easier to remember. "A universal compression-ventilation ratio (30:2) is recommended for all single rescuers of infant, child, and adult victims (excluding newborns)" [3]. To make CPR techniques easier for the lay rescuer to remember, some skills, such as rescue breathing, are not being taught to lay rescuers.

The guidelines state, "To be successful, CPR must be started as soon as a victim collapses, and we must therefore rely on a trained and willing public to initiate CPR and call for professional help and an AED [automated external defibrillator]. We have learned that when these steps happen in a timely manner, CPR makes a difference" [5].

After determining that the victim is unresponsive, the lay rescuer should telephone the emergency response number and obtain an automated external defibrillator (AED) or direct someone else to do so. The lay rescuer then should open the

airway and check for normal breathing and, if normal breathing is not present, give two initial breaths. After giving the initial two breaths, the lay rescuer is taught to begin cycles of 30 compressions and two ventilations immediately. The AED should be used as soon as it arrives. The lay rescuer is not taught to assess the unresponsive victim for a pulse or other signs of circulation.

The health care provider is taught to deviate from this response based on the most likely cause of the event. If the unresponsive victim collapsed suddenly, the health care provider either telephones the emergency response number and obtains an AED or directs someone else to do so. If alone, the health care provider leaves the victim to telephone the emergency response number and obtain the AED and then returns to the victim to address the airway/breath/circulation (ABC) concerns of CPR and to use the AED. The guidelines state, "For unresponsive victims of all ages with likely asphyxia arrest (eg, drowning) the lone health care provider should deliver about 5 cycles (about 2 minutes) of CPR before leaving the victim to telephone the emergency response number and get the AED" [3]. After telephoning the emergency response number and obtaining the AED, the rescuer returns to the victim to begin CPR and use the AED. The rescuer should open the airway and check for normal breathing and, if normal breathing is not present, give two initial breaths. After giving the initial two breaths, the health care provider spends no more than 10 seconds trying to feel a pulse. If no pulse is found within this 10-second period, the rescuer begins cycles of 30 compressions and two breaths.

Health care providers continue to be taught rescue breathing for the victim who has a pulse but either is not breathing or is making inadequate attempts to breathe (agonal gasps). If a pulse is found, but the victim is not breathing or is making inadequate attempts to breathe (agonal gasps), the health care provider provides rescue breathing (without chest compressions) at the rate of about one breath every 5 or 6 seconds for an adult (10–12 breaths per minute) or at the rate of one breath every 3 to 5 seconds for a child or infant (12–20 breaths per minute).

Once an advanced airway (endotracheal tube, laryngeal mask airway, or combined esophageal-tracheal tube [Combitube]) has been placed and its position confirmed, it is no longer necessary in two-rescuer CPR for rescuers to pause compressions for ventilations. The compressor continues to compress at a rate of 100 compressions per minute, and the ventilator provider gives a breath every 6 to 8 seconds (about 8–10 breaths per minute). To prevent fatigue, rescuers should change roles about every 2 minutes.

According to the guidelines, "Child CPR guidelines for the lay rescuer apply to children about 1 to 8 years of age, and adult guidelines for the lay rescuer apply to victims about 8 years of age and older" [6]. Furthermore, "Child CPR guidelines for health care providers apply to victims from about 1 year of age to the onset of adolescence or puberty (about 12 to 14 years of age) as defined by the presence of secondary sex characteristics" [6]. Infant CPR guidelines apply to infants younger than 1 year; infants are considered newborn within the first hours after birth, until they leave the hospital.

In children, the rescuer uses either one or two hands to compress the child's chest to a depth of one third to one half the depth of the chest, being careful to allow full recoil. Lay rescuers use a 30:2 ratio of compressions to ventilations. Health care providers use the 30:2 ratio when alone, but for two-rescuer CPR on a child victim, health care providers use a 15:2 ratio of compressions to ventilations.

Lay rescuers use two fingers just below the nipple line to compress the lower half of the infant's sternum with a 30:2 ratio of compressions to ventilations. The lone health care provider also uses two fingers just below the nipple line to compress the lower half of the infant's sternum with a 30:2 ratio of compressions to ventilations. When a second health care provider is present, the ratio changes to 15:2 compressions to ventilations, and the preferred technique is to use two thumbs with the hands encircling the infant's chest.

Defibrillation

The guidelines state, "Early defibrillation is critical to survival from sudden cardiac arrest (SCA) for several reasons: (1) the most frequent initial rhythm in witnessed SCA is ventricular fibrillation (VF), (2) the treatment for VF is electrical defibrillation, (3) the probability of successful defibrillation diminishes rapidly over time, and (4) VF tends to deteriorate to asystole within a few minutes" [7]. Rescuers must be able to integrate CPR with the use of the AED rapidly to treat ventricular fibrillation (VF) in sudden cardiac arrest. Three actions must occur within the first moments of a cardiac arrest to give the victim the best chance of survival: activation of Emergency Medical System (EMS), CPR, and use of an AED. Delays in CPR or defibrillation can reduce the chance of survival.

When an out-of-hospital arrest is witnessed, and an AED is on site, the rescuer should use the AED as soon as possible. If an in-hospital arrest occurs and an AED is on site, immediate CPR should be provided, and the AED/defibrillator should be used as soon as available. If an out-of-hospital arrest is not witnessed, EMS personnel may give about 2 minutes of CPR (approximately five cycles of 30 compressions to two ventilations) before checking the ECG rhythm and attempting defibrillation. In clinical studies, when the EMS response time was 4 to 5 minutes (or longer), the survival rate was higher for victims who were given 1.5 to 3 minutes of CPR before defibrillation. This protocol showed "an increased rate of initial resuscitation, survival to hospital discharge and 1 year survival when compared with those who received immediate defibrillation for VF SCA" [7].

A rhythm analysis of an AED's three-shock sequence showed a delay of up to 37 seconds between the delivery of the first shock and the first compression after shock. The guidelines state, "When VF/pulseless ventricular tachycardia (VT) is present, the rescuer should deliver 1 shock and should then immediately resume CPR, beginning with chest compressions (Class IIa)" [8]. Chest compressions should not be delayed to recheck the rhythm or pulse. CPR should be continued for five cycles (about 2 minutes) before the AED analyzes the rhythm and delivers another shock if indicated. The guidelines state, "If a nonshockable rhythm is detected, the AED should instruct the rescuer to resume CPR immediately, beginning with chest compressions (class IIb)" [8].

Monophasic waveform defibrillators deliver current with flow in one direction. According to the guidelines, "Biphasic defibrillators use one of two waveforms, and each waveform has been shown to be effective in terminating VF over a specific dose range. ... Current research confirms that it is reasonable to use selected energies of 150 J to 200 J with a biphasic truncated exponential waveform or 120 J with a rectilinear biphasic waveform for the initial shock" [9].

Studies of lay-rescuer AED programs have reported a survival rate of 41% to 74% in out-of-hospital, witnessed VF/sudden cardiac arrest when immediate bystander CPR is provided and defibrillation occurs within 3 to 5 minutes.

According to the guidelines [10], "The following elements are recommended for community lay rescuer AED programs:

- A planned and practiced response; typically this requires oversight by a health care provider
- Training of anticipated rescuers in CPR and use of the AED
- Link with the local EMS system
- Process of ongoing quality improvement"

If lay-rescuer AED programs are created in locations where sudden cardiac arrest is likely to occur, such as airports, sport facilities, and other public locations, they will have the greatest potential for increasing survival from sudden cardiac arrest. VF is seen in 5% to 15% of pediatric and adolescent arrests; when VF is present, rapid defibrillation may improve the outcome. The lowest amount of energy for effective defibrillation and the upper limit of energy for safe defibrillation are unknown, but doses greater than 4 J/kg have been used effectively to defibrillate children. The recommended energy dose to defibrillate children with either a monophasic or biphasic manual defibrillator is 2 J/kg for the first attempt, increased to 4 J/kg for subsequent attempts. Many AEDs can detect VF in children and distinguish between a shockable and a nonshockable rhythm. Some AEDs are equipped with a pediatric switch; others use pediatric pads that have an in-line reducer. If an AED does not have pediatric pads or a pediatric switch, the rescuer should use the standard AED but not allow the pads to touch. The pads may need to be placed in the anterior/posterior position on a very small child.

The guidelines advise, "If a provider is operating a manual biphasic defibrillator and is unaware of the effective dose range for that device to terminate VF, the rescuer may use a selected dose of 200 J for the first shock and an equal or higher dose for the second and subsequent shocks" [11]. If a monophasic defibrillator is used, a dose of 360 J is used for all shocks. Several factors, such as transthoracic impedance, electrode position, and electrode size, can affect defibrillation success. Conductive materials, such as gel pads, electrode paste, or self-adhesive pads, should be used to reduce transthoracic impedance. The contact between electrode and chest may be poor in a patient who has a hairy chest, and it may be necessary to shave the chest to allow better contact.

Pads or paddles should be well separated, and neither the pads nor the conductive materials should be touching. The pads should not be placed over or close to the device generator for permanent pacemakers or implantable cardio-defibrillators. The largest size electrode that can fit the chest without overlap should be used to decrease transthoracic impedance.

Cardiac arrest

The guidelines state, "The foundation of ACLS [advanced cardiac life-support] care is good BLS [basic life support] care, beginning with prompt high quality bystander CPR and, for VF/pulseless VT, attempted defibrillation within minutes of collapse" [12]. Comparatively, typical advanced cardiac life-support (ACLS) therapies have not shown an increase in the rate of survival to hospital discharge. Basic CPR and defibrillation are considered of primary importance during cardiac arrest. Because few drugs used in the treatment of cardiac arrest are supported by strong evidence, drug administration is considered of secondary importance. Peripheral intravenous sites are preferred because they do not require interruption of CPR for insertion. Resuscitation drugs administered through a peripheral site take longer to reach the central circulation; the drug should be followed by administration of a 20-mL intravenous fluid bolus along with elevation of the extremity for 10 to 20 seconds. Intraosseous insertion is a noncollapsible, safe, and effective route for delivery of fluids and drugs. Lidocaine, epinephrine, atropine, naloxone, and vasopressin can be administered by the endotracheal route if intravenous or intraosseous administration cannot be established, but lower blood concentrations can result. Administration of atropine and epinephrine by the intravenous route was associated with a higher rate of return of spontaneous circulation than seen with endotracheal administration. The optimal endotracheal drug dose is unknown, but diluting the recommended dose in 5 to 10 mL of water or normal saline is recommended before injecting the drug into the endotracheal tube.

The guidelines state, "When a rhythm check reveals VF/VT, rescuers should provide CPR while the defibrillator charges (when possible), until it is time to 'clear' the victim for shock delivery" [13]. The shock should be given as quickly as possible, and CPR should be resumed beginning with chest compressions. CPR should continue for 2 minutes before the rhythm is checked. The goal is to minimize the number of times chest compressions are interrupted. The Hs and Ts (Hypovolemia, Hypoxia, Hydrogenion (acidosis), Hypo/Hyperkalemia, Hypoglycemia, Hypothermia and Toxins, Tamponade (cardiac), Tension pneumothorax, Thrombosis (coronary or pulmonary), Trauma) should be reviewed to identify possible causes of the arrest or factors that may be complicating the situation. A vasopressor may be given if VF/VT persists after one or two shocks plus CPR, but CPR should not be interrupted to give medications. The drug should be given as soon as possible after the rhythm is checked and during CPR so that it can be circulated. Drugs can be administered either before or after the shock. Ideally, the guidelines state, the "drug doses should be prepared before the rhythm check so they can be administered as soon as possible after the rhythm check, but the timing of drug delivery is less important than the need to minimize interruptions in chest compressions" [13].

According to the guidelines, "Research with cardiac ultrasonography and indwelling pressure catheters has confirmed that pulseless patients with electrical activity have associated mechanical contractions, but these contractions are too weak to produce a blood pressure detectable by palpation or noninvasive blood pressure monitoring. PEA [pulseless electrical activity] is often caused by reversible conditions and can be treated if those conditions are identified and corrected" [14]. Asystole has a low survival rate. The hope for resuscitation lies in identifying and treating the cause of pulseless electrical activity or asystole. The focus is on performing high-quality CPR and identifying and treating reversible causes. Attempted pacing in asystole did not show benefit and is not recommended.

Symptomatic bradycardia and tachycardia

ACLS providers must take care to base their treatments on the whole clinical picture, not just on the presenting rhythm. The guidelines outline [15]: "The principles of arrhythmia recognition and management in adults are as follows:

- If bradycardia produces signs and symptoms (eg, acute altered mental status, ongoing severe ischemic chest pain, congestive heart failure, hypotension, or other signs of shock) that persist despite adequate airway and breathing, prepare to provide pacing. For symptomatic high-degree (second-degree or third-degree) atrioventricular (AV) block, provide transcutaneous pacing without delay.
- If the tachycardic patient is unstable with severe signs and symptoms related to tachycardia, prepare for immediate cardioversion.
- If the patient with tachycardia is unstable, determine if the patient has a narrow-complex or wide-complex tachycardia and then tailor therapy accordingly.
- You must understand the initial diagnostic electrical and drug treatment options for rhythms that are unstable or immediately life-threatening.
- Know when to call for expert consultation regarding complicated rhythm interpretation, drugs, or management decisions."

The initial treatment of bradycardia is to support the airway and breathing. One should provide supplementary oxygen, place the victim on the monitor, and obtain vital signs. One should determine whether signs and symptoms of poor perfusion are caused by the bradycardia. Asymptomatic patients should be monitored for deterioration. Atropine is the drug of choice for acute symptomatic bradycardia without reversible causes. For symptomatic high-degree block (second-degree or third-degree block), transcutaneous pacing should be used.

Most wide complex tachycardias are ventricular in origin. If the patient is unstable (shows signs and symptoms such as altered mental status, ongoing chest pain, hypotension, or other signs of shock), one should immediately deliver synchronized cardioversion (do not delay to administer drugs). If the patient is stable, one should obtain a 12-lead ECG and evaluate the rhythm to determine treatment. Synchronizing the shock during cardioversion allows the shock delivery to be timed with the QRS complex and avoids delivery during the relative refractory period of the cardiac cycle. Low-energy unsynchronized shocks may induce VF.

References

[1] AHA Web site. Facts about women and cardiovascular disease. Available at: www.americanheart.org/presenter.jhtml?identifer=2876. Accessed December 28, 2007.
[2] Center for Disease Control and Prevention's Web site. Sandmaier N. A healthy heart handbook for women. (NIH pub 07-2720). Available

at: www.nhlbi.nih.gov/health/public/heart/other/ hhw/hdbk_wmn.pdf. Accessed December 28, 2007.

[3] 2005 AHA Guidelines for CPR and ECC. Circulation 2005;112(24):IV–12.

[4] 2005 AHA Guidelines for CPR and ECC. Circulation 2005;112(24):IV–1.

[5] 2005 AHA Guidelines for CPR and ECC. Circulation 2005;112(24):IV–15.

[6] 2005 AHA Guidelines for CPR and ECC. Circulation 2005;112(24):IV–13.

[7] 2005 AHA Guidelines for CPR and ECC. Circulation 2005;112(24):IV–35.

[8] 2005 AHA Guidelines for CPR and ECC. Circulation 2005;112(24):IV–36.

[9] 2005 AHA Guidelines for CPR and ECC. Circulation 2005;112(24):IV–37.

[10] 2005 AHA Guidelines for CPR and ECC. Circulation 2005;112(24):IV–38.

[11] 2005 AHA Guidelines for CPR and ECC. Circulation 2005;112(24):IV–40.

[12] 2005 AHA Guidelines for CPR and ECC. Circulation 2005;112(24):IV–58.

[13] 2005 AHA Guidelines for CPR and ECC. Circulation 2005;112(24):IV–60.

[14] 2005 AHA Guidelines for CPR and ECC. Circulation 2005;112(24):IV–61.

[15] 2005 AHA Guidelines for CPR and ECC. Circulation 2005;112(24):IV–67.

ELSEVIER
SAUNDERS

Crit Care Nurs Clin N Am 20 (2008) 251–263

CRITICAL CARE
NURSING CLINICS
OF NORTH AMERICA

Raising Awareness of Women and Heart Disease—Women's Hearts are Different

Cheryl Herrmann, RN, MS, APN, CCRN, CCNS-CSC/CMC

Methodist Medical Center of Illinois, 221 NE. Glen Oak Avenue, Peoria, IL 61636, USA

Contrary to what many women believe, heart disease, not breast cancer, is the foremost killer of women. One of 2.6 women dies from cardiovascular disease (CVD) [1] compared with 1 in 30 who die of breast cancer. CVD is the leading single cause of death in all women worldwide [2,3]. With the exception of the influenza epidemic of 1918, heart disease has been the number one killer of both American men and women for more than 100 years. Mortality from CVD has decreased for men during the past 20 years but has remained essentially unchanged for women [1]. Heart disease is not just a man's disease; it is an equal opportunity killer.

Awareness

Women do not realize that heart disease is their greatest health risk. In 1990, a health care Gallup poll of more than 1000 women found that 46% believed their greatest health risk was breast cancer, and only 4% saw heart disease as their greatest risk. Statistically, in fact, 36% of these women would develop heart disease, and 4% would develop breast cancer [4]. Ten years later another survey found only 8% of American women considered heart disease and stroke as their greatest risk [5,6].

In response to the surveys several national awareness programs have been launched to raise awareness about women's risk for developing heart disease. Two of these programs are "The Heart Truth" and "Go for Red." "The Heart Truth" was introduced in 2003 with the First Lady, Laura Bush, serving as one of the Heart Truth's Ambassadors to help lead the campaign. The red dress was introduced as the national symbol for heart disease awareness for women at Fashion week 2003 [7]. The American Heart Association's "Go Red for Women. Love Your Heart" national movement began in February 2004 to encourage the public and health care professionals to pay attention to heart disease in women [8].

To evaluate trends in women's awareness, knowledge, and perceptions related to CVD since 1997, the American Heart Association (AHA) conducted another study in 2006. This study found that 57% women identified heart disease as the leading cause of death, but only 22% perceived heart disease as the greatest health problem among women. Even though women have become more aware that heart disease is the leading cause of death, they have not personalized this information [6]. This recent study does show the positive influence of the national programs to educate women about heart disease.

Women's heart guidelines

In 2004 the AHA published the first evidence–based guidelines for prevention of cardiovascular disease prevention in women [9]. These guidelines were updated in 2007 [3]. The 2004 guidelines emphasized the importance of heart disease and classified women into high, medium, low, and optimal risk groups based on the Framingham global risk score. The 2007 guidelines recommend a heart-healthy lifestyle and stratified risk categories as "high risk," "at risk," and "optimal risk" (Box 1). Given that the average lifetime risk for CVD in women is very high, approaching one in two, prevention is important for all women. With the 2004 guidelines, a 43-year-old woman

E-mail address: cherrmann@verizon.net

0899-5885/08/$ - see front matter © 2008 Elsevier Inc. All rights reserved.
doi:10.1016/j.ccell.2008.03.002

Box 1. Classification of the risk of cardiovascular disease (CVD) in women

High risk
Established coronary heart disease
Cerebrovascular disease
Peripheral arterial disease
Abdominal aortic aneurysm
End-stage or chronic renal disease
10-Year Framingham global risk > 20%[a]

At risk
One or more major risk factors for CVD, including
 • Cigarette smoking
 • Poor diet
 • Physical inactivity
 • Obesity, especially central adiposity
 • Family history of premature CVD (CVD at age < 55 years of age in a male relative or < 65 years of age in a female relative)
 • Hypertension
 • Dyslipidemia
Evidence of subclinical vascular disease (eg, coronary calcification)
Metabolic syndrome
Poor exercise capacity on treadmill test and/or abnormal heart rate recovery after stopping exercise

Optimal risk
Framingham global risk < 10% and a healthful lifestyle, with no risk factors.

_____
 [a] Or at high risk on the basis of another population-adapted tool used to assess global risk.
 Reprinted with permission from Evidence Based Guidelines for Cardiovascular Disease Prevention in Women: 2007 Update. © 2007, American Heart Association.

of premature CVD, dyslipidemia (as noted by the HDL cholesterol level of 42 mg/dL and non-HDL cholesterol level of 136 mg/dL) is classified as "at risk" for heart disease. The 2007 guidelines give specific recommendations on how to prevent heart disease [3]. These recommendations are discussed later in this article and are summarized in Appendices 1 and 2. The levels of evidence are listed in Box 2.

Understanding cardiovascular risks

Risk factors

The risk factors for heart disease in women can be categorized as nonmodifiable or modifiable.

Nonmodifiable risk factors
Nonmodifiable risk factors are age and a positive family history for premature CVD.

Positive family history. A positive family history of premature CVD is CVD in a male relative younger than 55 years of age or in a female relative younger than 65 years. Knowing the

Box 2. Classification and levels of evidence: strength of recommendation

Classification
Class I: Intervention is useful and effective.
Class IIa: Weight of evidence/opinion is in favor of usefulness/efficacy.
Class IIb: Usefulness/efficacy is less well established by evidence/opinion.
Class III: Intervention is not useful/ effective and may be harmful.

Level of evidence
A: Sufficient evidence from multiple randomized trials
B: Limited evidence from a single randomized trial or other nonrandomized studies
C: Based on expert opinion, case studies, or standard of care

_____
 Reprinted with permission from Evidence Based Guidelines for Cardiovascular Disease Prevention in Women: 2007 Update. © 2007, American Heart Association.

who does not smoke, who has a total cholesterol level of 178 mg/dL, a high-density lipoprotein (HDL) cholesterol level of 42 mg/dL, and blood pressure of 122/86 has a probability, according to the Framingham 10-year risk score, of having the coronary event by age 53 years of less than 1% and is classified as low risk. With the 2007 guidelines this same woman, who also has the risk factors of central obesity, a family history family history can help to motivate individuals to reduce other risk factors and help health care providers stratify risk.

Age. Women age 55 years and older are at risk for CVD. Before menopause, estrogen helps protect women from CVD by increasing HDL cholesterol, lowering low-density (LDL) cholesterol, antiplatelet effects, and reduction of angiotensin-converting enzyme activity, so women typically are 10 years older than men when they develop CVD. With increasing age, increasing comorbidities increase a woman's risk. The average age at which women have a first acute myocardial infarction (AMI) is 70.4 years, compared with 65.8 years for men [1].

In the 1990s it was recommended that women use hormone replacement therapy to protect against heart disease, because it was thought that the benefits outweighed the risks [10]. It later was realized that the risks of hormone replacement therapy (deep vein thrombosis/pulmonary embolism, breast cancer, stroke, dementia) outweigh the benefits. Hormone replacement therapy may be used for treatment of menopausal symptoms but should not be used for prevention of CVD [11]. The AHA recommendation (class III, level A) is that hormone therapy and selective estrogen-receptor modulators should not be used for the primary or secondary prevention of CVD.

Modifiable risk factors

Smoking, hypertension, diabetes, poor diet, sedentary lifestyle, and obesity are risk factors for heart disease in women that can be modified.

Smoking. Smoking is the greatest preventable cause of death in the United States. The risk of heart attack is up to six times greater for women whom smoke than for women who do not smoke [1]. Cigarette smokers are two to four times more likely than nonsmokers to develop CVD. Smoking causes vasoconstriction of the arteries, and toxins in the blood from cigarette smoking contribute to the development of atherosclerosis [12]. Women face special barriers to quitting smoking, such as concerns about weight gain and concomitant depression.

Recommendations of the American Heart Association. The recommendations of the AHA are that women should not smoke and should avoid environmental tobacco smoke (class I, level B). One should provide counseling, nicotine replacement, and other pharmacotherapy as indicated in conjunction with a behavioral program or a formal smoking cessation program.

Diabetes. Diabetes affects 8.8% of women over the age of 20 years [13]. The prevalence of diabetes increases with age; 21% of adults older than 60 years have diabetes. The median age at which women are diagnosed with diabetes decreased by 6.7 years between 1980 (58.4 years) and 2005 (51.7 years) [13]. Diabetes rates continue to escalate, as indicated in the diabetes trend maps in Fig. 1 [14]. Latinas, American Indian, African American, Asian American, and Pacific Islander women are at a higher risk than white American women for diabetes. The death rates from heart disease are two to four times higher among women who have diabetes than among women who do not have diabetes [1]. At least 65% of people who have diabetes mellitus die of some form of heart disease or stroke [1]. Women who have diabetes often have high blood pressure, elevated cholesterol levels, and are overweight, factors that increase their risk even more.

Recommendations of the American Heart Association. Lifestyle and pharmacotherapy should be used as indicated in women who have diabetes (class I, level B) to achieve a hemoglobin A_{1C} below 7% (class I, level C).

Hypertension. Hypertension is defined as blood pressure greater than 140 to 159/90 to 99 mm Hg, and prehypertension is defined as blood pressure of 120 to 139/80 to 89 mm Hg [15]. Thirty-two percent of women in the United States have hypertension. For every 20 mm Hg systolic or 10 mm Hg diastolic increase in blood pressure, the risk of mortality from CVD doubles. African Americans develop hypertension earlier in life, have much higher average blood pressures, and have a 1.5 times greater risk of cardiac death than white Americans [1].

The lifestyle approaches to hypertension of the Joint National Committee for Prevention, Detection, Evaluation, and Treatment of High Blood Pressure are to maintain an ideal body weight, to follow the Dietary Approaches to Stop Hypertension eating plan, to increase physical activity, to use alcohol in moderation, and to restrict sodium to 2400 mg/d. Further reduction of sodium to 1500 mg/d may be beneficial, especially for African American women [15].

Recommendations of the American Heart Association. Control blood pressure through optimal level and lifestyle: encourage an optimal blood

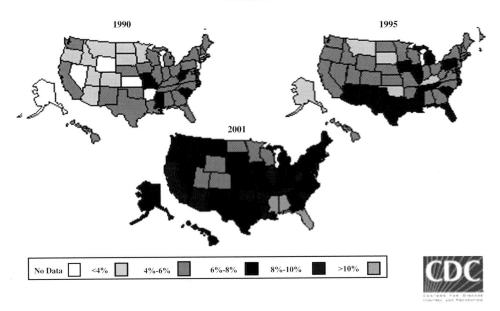

Fig. 1. Diabetes and gestational diabetes trends in adults in the United States. Behavioral Risk Factor Surveillance System, 1990, 1995, and 2001. (*Courtesy of* the Centers for Disease Control and Prevention, Atlanta, GA.)

pressure lower than 120/80 mm Hg through lifestyle approaches such as weight control, increased physical activity, alcohol moderation, sodium restriction, and increased consumption of fresh fruits, vegetables, and low-fat dairy products (class I, level B).

Pharmacotherapy for blood pressure: Pharmacotherapy is indicated when blood pressure is 140/90 mm Hg or higher or at a lower blood pressure ($\geq$ 130/80 mm Hg) in the setting of chronic kidney disease or diabetes. Thiazide diuretics should be part of the drug regimen for most patients unless they are contraindicated or there are compelling indications for using other agents in specific vascular diseases. Initial treatment of high-risk women should be with beta-blockers and/or angiotensin-converting enzyme inhibitors/angiotensin receptor blockers, with addition of other drugs such as thiazides as needed to achieve the target blood pressure (class I, level A).

Dyslipidemia. Dyslipidemia is defined as elevated LDL cholesterol, low HDL cholesterol, elevated total cholesterol, and elevated triglyceride levels. The optimal lipid and lipoprotein levels are LDL cholesterol below 100 mg/dL, HDL cholesterol above 50 mg/dL, triglycerides below 150 mg/dL, and non-HDL cholesterol (total cholesterol minus HDL cholesterol) below 130 mg/dL (class I, level A) [3], and total cholesterol below 200 mg/dL [16].

For many years public education emphasized keeping total cholesterol below 200 mg/dL, and little attention was given to HDL cholesterol. HDL cholesterol ("happy cholesterol") plays an important role in protection against CVD. For every 1-mg/dL increase in HDL cholesterol, there is a 3% decrease in CVD risk for women. A low HDL cholesterol level is of greater concern in women than in men [17]. The total cholesterol/HDL cholesterol ratio is another way to evaluate the risk of CVD and is very predictive of risk in women. The total cholesterol/HDL ratio is obtained by dividing the total cholesterol by the HDL cholesterol. A ratio less than 2.5 suggests below-average risk for CVD, a ratio of 2.9 to 4.0 indicates average risk, and a ratio greater than 4.0 indicates above-average risk. The non-HDL cholesterol (total cholesterol minus HDL cholesterol) should be less than 130 mg/dL.

In Table 1, woman A, who is 40 years old, has a total cholesterol less than 200 mg/dL. The total cholesterol could give a false sense of security if one does not consider the other lipoprotein values. Based on her total cholesterol/HDL cholesterol ratio of 4.5, non-HDL cholesterol level greater than 130, and low HDL cholesterol level, this woman has an above-average risk for CVD. Based only on total cholesterol, Woman B, who is 70 years old, would seem to be at higher risk than woman A. When all lipoprotein values are

Table 1
Examples of cholesterol and lipoprotein

Characteristic	Woman A	Woman B
Age (female)	40 years	70 years
Total cholesterol	178 mg/dL	257 mg/dL
Low-density lipoprotein cholesterol	113 mg/dL	167 mg/dL
High-density lipoprotein cholesterol	40 mg/dL	63 mg/dL
Ratio	4.5	4.1
Non-high-density lipoprotein cholesterol	138 mg/dL	194 mg/dL
Triglycerides	124 mg/dL	135 mg/dL

considered, however, Woman A is at greater lifetime risk for a cardiac event, especially because she is only 40 years old, whereas Woman B is 70 years old and has no cardiac history.

Elevated triglycerides usually are related to lifestyle (overweight, smoking, sedentary lifestyle, diet high in carbohydrates) and often correlate with high total cholesterol levels. Triglyceride elevation has greater atherogenic significance in women than in men.

Recommendations. Appendix 1 gives lifestyle approaches and pharmacologic for obtaining optimal lipid levels.

Poor diet, sedentary lifestyle, and obesity. Poor diet, sedentary lifestyle, and obesity (body mass index greater than 30) [18] are listed together because the risk factors of poor diet and a sedentary lifestyle tend to lead to obesity. All three risk factors increase the risk of developing the other risk factors of dyslipidemia, hypertension, and diabetes. During the past 20 years there has been a dramatic increase in obesity among Americans, who are living in a "super size" society. The obesity trends noted when comparing the 1990 and 2006 data of the Center for Disease Control's Behavioral Risk Factor Surveillance System are alarming. In 1990, the prevalence of obesity was less than 10% in 10 states; by 1998, no state had a prevalence of less than 10%. In 1990, in no states was the prevalence of obesity 15% or higher, whereas in 2006, the prevalence of obesity was less than 20% in only four states. In 2006, the prevalence of obesity was 25% or higher in 22 states. In two of these states, Mississippi and West Virginia, the prevalence of obesity was 30% or higher (Fig. 2) [18].

The distribution of body fat is important in the risk for heart disease. Apple-shaped obesity or central obesity (with the bulk of fat around the waist/abdomen) is associated with a higher risk of heart disease than pear-shaped obesity (with the bulk of fat in the hips and thighs).

Contributing to the obesity epidemic are poor diet and sedentary lifestyle. A person eating 2000 calories should consume less than 65 g of fat and less than 2400 mg sodium [19]. To put these numbers in perspective, stopping at a fast-food restaurant on the way home from work and ordering a quarter-pound pound

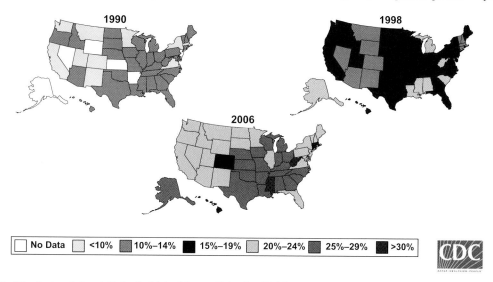

Fig. 2. Obesity trends in adults in the United States. Behavioral Risk Factor Surveillance System, 1990, 1998, and 2006. (Percent of population with BMI > 30 or about 30 pounds overweight for a 5′4″ person.) (*Courtesy of* the Centers for Disease Control and Prevention, Atlanta, GA.)

cheeseburger, a large serving of fries, and a medium-sized soft drink provides 1280 calories, 56 g of fat, and 1520 mg sodium for one meal [20]. What happens when the server asks, "Would you like to make that supersize?" The National Heart Lung and Blood Institute has recognized that food portions have increased in the last 20 years, resulting in larger waistlines and heavier body weights. Many portions are enough to feed two people. To increase awareness a "Portion Distortion" slide show can be downloaded to show the increase in food portions and the amount of exercise needed to burn off the extra food [21]. A meal consisting of a cheeseburger, fries, and soda in today's portions has 822 more calories than the same meal 20 years ago. One would need to exercise 3.25 hours to burn off the extra calories. Even with healthier choices, the larger portions still add more calories. For example, a chicken Caesar salad portion is 2 cups more and has 400 more calories than 20 years ago, and a turkey sandwich is has 500 more calories (Table 2).

In 2002, the Institute of Medicine and National Academies of Science reported that that *trans*-fatty acids increase LDL cholesterol ("bad cholesterol") and lower HDL cholesterol ("good cholesterol") in the blood, thereby increasing the risk of coronary heart disease [22]. *Trans* fat can be found in some of the foods that contain saturated fat, such as vegetable shortenings, some margarines, crackers, candies, cookies, snack foods, fried foods, baked goods, and other processed foods made with partially hydrogenated vegetable oils.

Thirty percent of women report having no leisure-time physical activity. African American and Hispanic women have the lowest prevalence of leisure time spent in physical activity [1]. The relative risk of CVD associated with physical inactivity ranges from 1.5 to 2.4, an increase in risk comparable to that observed for high cholesterol levels, high blood pressure, or cigarette smoking [23]. Walking briskly for 3 hours a week or exercising vigorously for 1.5 hours a week will reduce the risk of coronary heart disease in women by 30% to 40% [24]. To increase compliance with physical activity, the AHA has designed a free, 12-week "Choose to Move" physical activity program dedicated to helping women incorporate health-promoting habits into their existing routines. It focuses on practical ways women can reduce their risk for heart disease and stroke by increasing physical activity and eating healthful foods [25].

Recommendations. Weight maintenance/reduction: Women should maintain or lose weight through an appropriate balance of physical activity, caloric intake, and formal behavioral programs when indicated to maintain/achieve a body mass index between 18.5 and 24.9 and a waist circumference of 35 inches or more (class I, level B).

Dietary intake: Women should consume a diet rich in fruits and vegetables, choose whole-grain, high-fiber foods; eat fish, especially oily fish, at lease twice a week; limit intake of saturated fat to less than 10% of calories (and if possible to less than 7%), limit cholesterol to less than 300 mg/d, limit alcohol intake to no more than one drink per day, and limit sodium intake to less than 2.3 g/d (approximately 1 teaspoon of salt). Consumption of *trans*-fatty acids should be as low as possible (ie, < 1% of calories/energy) (class I, level B).

Table 2
Food distortion: how food portions have changed in the last 20 years

Food	Increase in calories in the last 20 years	Amount of exercise to burn off the extra calories
Bagel	210	50 minutes of raking leaves (130-lb person)
Cheeseburger	257	1.5 hours of lifting weights (130-lb person)
French fries	400	1.3 hours of walking (160-lb person)
Soda	165	35 minutes of garden work (160-lb person)
Spaghetti and meatballs	525	2 hours & 25 minutes of housecleaning (130-lb person)
Turkey sandwich	500	1 hour and 25 minutes of biking (160-lb person)
Coffee	305	1.3 hours of walking (130-lb person)
Caesar salad	400	1.3 hours of walking (160-lb person)
Popcorn	360	1.25 hours of water aerobics (160-lb person)
Chicken stir fry	460	1.1 hours of aerobic dancing (130-lb person)

Data from National Heart Lung and Blood Institute Food Portion Web site. Available at: http://hp2010.nhlbihin.net/portion/. Accessed November 7, 2007.

Omega-3 fatty acids: As an adjunct to diet, omega-3 fatty acids in capsule form (approximately 850–1000 mg of eicosapentaenoic acid and docosahexaenoic acid) may be considered in women who have CVD, and higher doses (2–4 g) may be used for treatment of women who have high triglyceride levels (class IIb, level B).

Physical activity: Women should accumulate a minimum of 30 minutes of moderate-intensity physical activity (ie, brisk walking) on most, and preferably all, days of the week (class I, level B).

Women who need to lose weight or sustain weight loss should accumulate a minimum of 60 to 90 minutes of moderate-intensity physical activity (ie, brisk walking) on most, and preferably all, days of the week (class I, level C).

Metabolic syndrome. Metabolic syndrome, a constellation of multiple interrelated risk factors, increases the risk for atherosclerotic CVD by 1.5- to threefold and raises the risk for type 2 diabetes by three- to fivefold. It affects more than 26% of adults, or more than 50 million Americans [16]. The hallmarks of metabolic syndrome in women are (1) abdominal obesity (waist circumference greater than 35 inches), (2) a triglyceride level of 150 mg/dL or higher, (3) a low HDL cholesterol level (< 50 mg/dL), (4) blood pressure higher than 130/85, and (5) fasting glucose level of 100 mg/dL or higher. Any three of the five criteria constitute a diagnosis of metabolic syndrome [1].

Recommendations. Lifestyle modification (as listed in each risk category) is the first-line therapy. Drug therapy may need to be added.

Risk assessment and stratification

The 2007 update of the AHA guidelines recommends the use of a scheme that classifies a woman as being at high risk, at risk, or at optimal risk (see Box 1). This risk stratification scheme places greater emphasis on lifetime risk than on short-term absolute risk [3]. A woman at high risk is one who has a history of coronary heart disease, cerebrovascular disease, peripheral arterial disease, abdominal aortic aneurysm, end-stage or chronic renal failure, or diabetes mellitus, and a 10-year Framingham global risk greater than 20%. A woman at risk is one who has more than one major risk factor for CVD, evidence of subclinical vascular disease, metabolic syndrome, and poor exercise capacity on treadmill test and/or abnormal heart rate recovery after stopping exercise. A woman at optimal risk is one who has a Framingham global risk of less than 10% and a healthful lifestyle, with no risk factors. The goal is for all women to be at their optimal risk. The Framingham point score [9] is an estimate of the likelihood that a woman will develop CVD within 10 years. It is calculated by giving points to the following risk factors: diabetes, age, smoking, total cholesterol, HDL cholesterol, and blood pressure. It does not include family history. The optimal-risk category can be used as a benchmark to motivate women to optimize modifiable risks and to live a health-inducing lifestyle. To help the health care practitioner in evaluating and prioritizing preventive interventions, a CVD preventive care in women algorithm is available in the 2007 update. The algorithm lists the class I and class II recommendations based on the woman's risks (Fig. 3).

Symptoms

The complexity and vagueness of symptoms in women make it difficult for a woman to recognize that she is having an AMI and for health care providers to diagnose and treat the AMI rapidly. Women may not experience the typical male AMI symptoms of "crushing chest pain radiating down the arms and to the jaw" but may have atypical chest pain consisting of chest discomfort, heaviness, tightness, or indigestion not related to something they ate, or they may not report any chest pain [26]. McSweeney and colleagues [27] found that only 29.7% of women who had an AMI reported having chest discomfort. Shortness of breath, extreme fatigue, and weakness are typical symptoms that many women report with AMI. McSweeney and colleagues [27] also found that 90% of women experienced prodromal symptoms, including unusual fatigue, sleep disturbances, shortness of breath, indigestion, and anxiety, before the development of AMI. African Americans women did not report chest pain but experienced shortness of breath, weakness, and dizziness with AMI [28].

The onset of clinical manifestations of CVD for women lags about 10 years behind men [29] and by 20 years for more serious events such as myocardial infarction and sudden death [1]. The older age of onset in women makes them more likely to have comorbidities such as hypertension, diabetes mellitus, and heart failure with preserved systolic function [30].

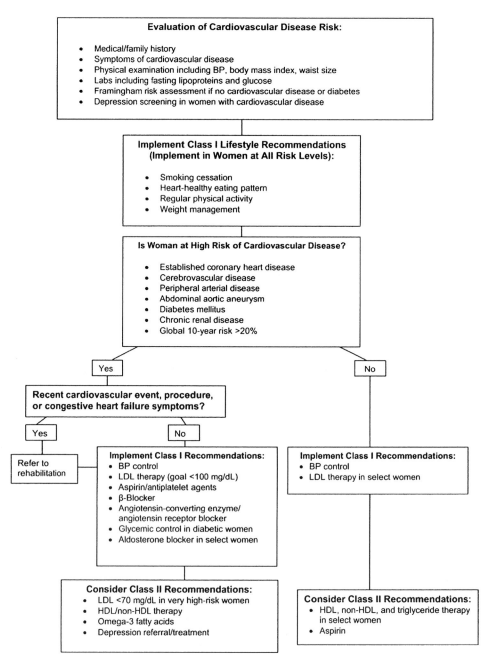

Fig. 3. Evaluation of the risk of cardiovascular disease in women. CVD, cardiovascular disease; HDL, high-density lipoprotein; LDL, low-density lipoprotein. (*Reprinted with permission from* Evidence Based Guidelines for Cardiovascular Disease Prevention in Women: 2007 Update. © 2007, American Heart Association.)

Delay in seeking treatment

To prevent damage to the heart muscle as much as possible and to decrease mortality, and morbidity, reperfusion treatment for an AMI must occur within a narrow time frame. Reperfusion within 90 minutes of onset of ischemia salvages about half of the myocardium at risk. Four to 6 hours after ischemia, salvage of the myocardium at risk is minimal [31]. The average patient who has ST segment elevation myocardial infarction (STEMI) waits approximately 2 hours after onset of symptoms to seek medical treatment, and women delay seeking treatment longer than men [31]. Women delay seeking treatment for AMI 1 to 6 hours longer than men [32]. Some of the reasons for delay can be the atypical presentation, lack of knowledge that women can have heart attacks, and other disease processes that have similar symptoms.

Every minute of delay in treatment of patients who have STEMI affects 1-year mortality. In fact, Giuseppe and colleagues [33] found that the risk of 1-year mortality for both men and women increased by 7.5% for each 30-minute delay in opening the artery with angioplasty. Because of their atypical symptoms and delay in seeking treatment, women should receive more education about heart disease to hasten treatment time and improve outcomes.

Diagnostic testing

Even though the guidelines for noninvasive testing in women are the same as in men, ECG stress exercise testing is less predictive in women than in men, primarily because of the lower pretest probability of coronary artery disease in women and a higher false-positive rate. With newer tissue software, however, breast attenuation artifact is less of a problem than previously with thallium-201 exercise testing. Dobutamine or exercise stress testing is an accurate and cost-effective technique for detecting coronary artery disease in women [30]. Clinical variables and risk factors need to be integrated into the diagnostic decision-making process. Women who have new-onset or rapidly worsening symptoms should be referred to an emergency department immediately for evaluation.

Cardiovascular research in women

Before 1990, women were underrepresented in controlled, randomized trials. In 1993, the National Institutes of Health Revitalization Act issued guidelines for women to be included in clinical trials [33]. Although the percentage of women included in trials increased from 20% between 1966 and 1990 to 25% between 1991 and 2000, women still are underrepresented in clinical studies [34]. The safety and efficacy of medications and treatments can vary, depending on the patient's sex and age, so research findings in younger

male cardiac patients may not be generalizable to older female cardiac patients.

Prognosis and treatment outcomes

Women tend to have worse clinical outcomes than men after coronary events and receive fewer treatments such as thrombolytics, percutaneous coronary interventions, and coronary artery bypass grafts (CABG), as shown by the following statistics:

- after AMI the mortality rate in women younger than 65 years is twice that of men of comparable age [1].
- Thirty-eight percent of women die within the first year after AMI, compared with 25% of men [1].
- Thirty-five percent of women have a second AMI within 6 years after the first AMI, compared with 18% of men [1].
- Forty-eight percent of women who have an AMI will be disabled with heart failure within 6 years after the AMI, compared with 22% of men [1].
- Women have more depression and physical disabilities after AMI [1].
- Mortality after CABG for women is double that in men. Women less than 50 years old undergoing CABG have three times the mortality rate of men of that age [1].
- Women have higher readmission rates and lower functional gains at 6 months after CABG than do men [35].
- Women have more anginal symptoms than men after percutaneous coronary interventions, resulting in more physical limitations and decreased quality of life [29].
- Women have more bleeding problems after thrombolysis, percutaneous coronary interventions, and CABG [29].
- Participation rates for eligible women in cardiac rehabilitation are 15% to 20%, compared with 25% to 31% for eligible men. Women are less likely to be encouraged to attend cardiac rehabilitation programs by health care providers and are more likely to drop out after beginning cardiac rehabilitation [36].

The higher risk profile (older age, more comorbidities, longer delays to treatment) often is given to explain these differences in outcomes [37]. Other explanations are the smaller coronary arteries in women; more urgent and emergent presentations; less frequent use of cholesterol screening and lipid-lowering treatments; less use of heparin, beta-blockers, and aspirin after AMI; less reperfusion therapy and angiography; and fewer referrals to cardiac rehabilitation [26].

In summary, a woman has a one-in-two lifetime risk of dying from a coronary event. Women and health care providers need to take action to understand the impact of coronary heart disease on women and to identify risk factors and implement the recommendations to help every woman be at optimal risk and to decrease the mortality from cardiac disease.

Acknowledgments

The author gratefully acknowledges the contributions of Melissa Hudak, MLIS, Library Services Coordinator, for the many reference searches and Susan Ripper, RN, CCRN for manuscript mentoring.

Appendix 1

Guidelines for prevention of cardiovascular disease in women: clinical recommendations

Lifestyle interventions

Cigarette smoking: Women should not smoke and should avoid environmental tobacco smoke. Provide counseling, nicotine replacement, and other pharmacotherapy as indicated in conjunction with a behavioral program or formal smoking cessation program (Class I, Level B).

Physical activity: Women should accumulate a minimum of 30 minutes of moderate-intensity physical activity (eg, brisk walking) on most, and preferably all, days of the week (Class I, Level B).

Women who need to lose weight or sustain weight loss should accumulate a minimum of 60 to 90 minutes of moderate-intensity physical activity (eg, brisk walking) on most, and preferably all, days of the week (Class I, Level C).

Rehabilitation: A comprehensive risk-reduction regimen, such as cardiovascular or stroke rehabilitation or a physician-guided home- or community-based exercise training program, should be recommended to women who have had a recent acute coronary syndrome or coronary intervention, new-onset or chronic angina, recent cerebrovascular event, peripheral arterial disease (Class I, Level A), or current/prior symptoms of heart failure and a left ventricular ejection fraction (LVEF) below 40% (Class I, Level B).

Dietary intake: Women should consume a diet rich in fruits and vegetables, choose whole-grain, high-fiber foods; consume fish, especially oily fish[a] at least twice a week; limit intake of saturated fat to less than 10% of energy, and if possible to less than 7%, cholesterol to less than 300 mg/d, alcohol intake to no more than one drink per day,[b] and sodium intake to less than 2.3 g/d (approximately 1 teaspoon salt). Consumption of *trans*-fatty acids should be as low as possible (eg, <1% of energy) (Class I, Level B).

Weight maintenance/reduction: Women should maintain or lose weight through an appropriate balance of physical activity, caloric intake, and formal behavioral programs when indicated to maintain/achieve a body mass index between 18.5 and 24.9 and a waist circumference of 35 inches or less (Class I, Level B).

Omega-3 fatty acids: As an adjunct to diet, omega-3 fatty acids in capsule form (approximately 850–1000 mg of of eicosapentaenoic acid and docosahexaenoic acid) may be considered in women who have coronary heart disease, and higher doses (2–4 g) may be used for treatment of women who have high triglyceride levels (Class IIb, Level B).

Depression: Consider screening women who have coronary heart disease for depression and refer/treat when indicated (Class IIa, Level B).

Major risk factor interventions

Blood pressure: optimal level and lifestyle. Encourage an optimal blood pressure below 120/80 mm Hg through lifestyle approaches such as weight control, increased physical activity, alcohol moderation, sodium restriction, and increased consumption of fresh fruits, vegetables, and low-fat dairy products (Class I, Level B).

Blood pressure: pharmacotherapy. Pharmacotherapy is indicated when blood pressure is 140/90 mm Hg or higher or at an even lower blood pressure ((≥ 130/80 mm Hg) in the setting of chronic kidney disease or diabetes. Thiazide diuretics should be part of the drug regimen for most patients unless contraindicated or there are compelling indications for other agents in specific vascular diseases. Initial treatment of high-risk women[c] should be with beta-blockers and/or angiotensin-converting enzyme (ACE) inhibitors/angiotensin receptor blockers (ARBs), with addition of other drugs such as thiazides as needed to achieve goal blood pressure (Class I, Level A).

Lipid and lipoprotein levels: optimal levels and lifestyle. The following levels of lipids and lipoproteins in women should be encouraged through lifestyle approaches: LDL cholesterol less than 100 mg/dL; HDL cholesterol more than 50 mg/dL; triglycerides lower than 150 mg/dL; and non-HDL cholesterol (total cholesterol minus HDL cholesterol) less than 130 mg/dL (Class I, Level B). If a woman is at high risk[c] or has hypercholesterolemia, intake of saturated fat should be less than 7% of total calories, and cholesterol intake should be less than 200 mg/d) (Class I, Level B).

Lipids: pharmacotherapy for lowering LDL in high-risk women.

Use LDL cholesterol–lowering drug therapy simultaneously with lifestyle therapy in women who have coronary heart disease to achieve an LDL cholesterol level lower than 100 mg/dL (Class I, Level A) and similarly in women who have other atherosclerotic CVD, diabetes mellitus, or a 10-year absolute risk greater than 20% (Class I, Level B).

A reduction to less than 70 mg/dL is reasonable in very high-risk women[d] who have coronary heart disease and may require an LDL-lowering drug combination (Class IIa, Level B).

Lipids: pharmacotherapy for lowering LDL in other at-risk women.

Use LDL cholesterol–lowering therapy if the LDL cholesterol level is 130 mg/dL or higher with lifestyle therapy and there are multiple risk factors and 10-year absolute risk of 10% to 20% (Class I, Level B).

Use LDL cholesterol–lowering therapy if the LDL cholesterol level is 160 mg/dL or higher with lifestyle therapy and there are and multiple risk factors, even if the 10-year absolute risk is less than 10% (Class I, Level B).

Use LDL cholesterol–lowering therapy if the LDL cholesterol level is 190 mg/dL with lifestyle therapy regardless of the presence or absence of other risk factors or CVD (Class I, Level B).

Lipids: pharmacotherapy for low HDL cholesterol or elevated non-HDL cholesterol in high-risk women. Use niacin or fibrate therapy when HDL cholesterol is low or non-HDL cholesterol is elevated in high-risk women after LDL cholesterol goal is reached (Class IIa, Level B).

Lipids: pharmacotherapy for low HDL or elevated non-HDL cholesterol in other at-risk women. Consider niacin[e] or fibrate therapy when HDL cholesterol is low or non-HDL cholesterol is elevated after LDL cholesterol goal is reached in women who have multiple risk factors and a 10-year absolute risk of 10% to 20% (Class IIb, Level B).

Diabetes mellitus: Lifestyle and pharmacotherapy should be used as indicated in women who have diabetes (Class I, Level B) to achieve a hemoglobinn A_{1c} below 7%, if this can be accomplished without significant hypoglycemia (Class I, Level C).

Preventive drug interventions

Aspirin: high-risk women. Aspirin therapy (75–325 mg/d)[f] should be used in high-risk[c] women unless contraindicated (Class I, Level A).

If a high-risk[c] woman is intolerant of aspirin therapy, clopidogrel should be substituted (Class I, Level B).

Aspirin: other at-risk or healthy women. In women 65 years of age or older, consider aspirin therapy (81 mg daily or 100 mg every other day) if blood pressure is controlled and the benefit for preventing ischemic stroke and myocardial infarction is likely to outweigh the risk of gastrointestinal bleeding and hemorrhagic stroke (Class IIa, Level B) and in women younger than 65 years when the benefit for preventing ischemic stroke is likely to outweigh the adverse effects of therapy (Class IIb, Level B).

Beta-blockers: Beta-blockers should be used indefinitely in all women after a myocardial infarction, acute coronary syndrome, or left ventricular dysfunction with or without heart failure symptoms, unless contraindicated (Class I, Level A).

ACE inhibitors/ARBs: ACE inhibitors should be used (unless contraindicated) in women who have had a myocardial infarction and in those who have clinical evidence of heart failure or an left LVEF of 40% or more or who have diabetes mellitus (Class I, Level A). ARBs should be used instead of ACE inhibitors in women who have had a myocardial infarction and in those who have clinical evidence of heart failure or an LVEF of

40% or more or who have diabetes mellitus who are intolerant of ACE inhibitors (Class I, Level B).

Aldosterone blockade: Use aldosterone blockade after a myocardial infarction in women who do not have significant renal dysfunction or hyperkalemia who already are receiving therapeutic doses of an ACE inhibitor and a beta-blocker and who have symptomatic heart failure with an LVEF of 40% or less (Class I, Level B).

[a] Pregnant and lactating women should avoid eating fish potentially high in methylmercury (eg, shark, swordfish, king mackerel, or tile fish). They should eat up to 12 ounces/week of a variety of fish and shellfish low in mercury. They should check the Environmental Protection Agency and the US Food and Drug Administration's Web sites for updates and local advisories about safety of local catch.

[b] One drink of alcohol is equivalent is equal to a 12-ounce bottle of beer, a 5-ounce glass of wine, or a 1.5-ounce shot of 80-proof spirits.

[c] Criteria for high risk include established coronary heart diseases, cerebrovascular disease, peripheral arterial disease, abdominal aortic aneurysm, end-stage or chronic renal disease, diabetes mellitus, and a 10-year Framingham risk greater than 20%.

[d] Criteria for very high risk include established CVD plus any of the following: multiple major risk factors, severe and poorly controlled risk factors, diabetes mellitus.

[e] Dietary supplement niacin should not be used as a substitute for prescription niacin.

[f] After percutaneous intervention with stent placement or coronary artery bypass grafting within the previous year and in women who have non-coronary forms of CVD, use current guidelines for aspirin and clopidogrel.

(*Reprinted with permission from* Evidence Based Guidelines for Cardiovascular Disease Prevention in Women: 2007 Update. © 2007, American Heart Association.)

Appendix 2

Class III interventions (not useful/effective and may be harmful) for cardiovascular disease or myocardial infarction prevention in women

Menopausal therapy: Hormone therapy and selective estrogen-receptor modulators should not be used for the primary or secondary prevention of CVD (Class III, Level A).

Antioxidant supplements: Antioxidant vitamin supplements (eg, vitamins E, C, and beta-carotene) should not be used for the primary or secondary prevention of CVD (Class III, Level A).

Folic acid[a]: Folic acid, with or without vitamin B_6 and vitamin B_{12} supplementation, should not be used for the primary or secondary prevention of CVD (Class III, Level A).

Aspirin for myocardial infarction in women younger than 65 years of age[b]: Routine use of aspirin to prevent myocardial infarction in healthy women younger than 65 years of age is not recommended (Class III, Level B).

[a] Folic acid supplementation should be used in the childbearing years to prevent neural tube defects.

[b] For recommendations for aspirin to prevent CVD in women age 65 years or older or stroke in women younger than 65 years, please see Appendix 1.

(*Reprinted with permission from* Evidence Based Guidelines for Cardiovascular Disease Prevention in Women: 2007 Update. © 2007, American Heart Association.)

References

[1] American Heart Association. Heart disease and stroke statistics—2007 update. Dallas (TX): American Heart Association; 2007.

[2] World Heart Federation. Available at: http://www.world-heart-federation.org/what-we-do/go-red-for-women/. Accessed November 7, 2007.

[3] Mosca L, Banka C, Benjamin E, et al. Evidence-based guidelines for cardiovascular disease prevention in women: 2007 update. Circulation 2007;115:1481–501.

[4] National Center for Health Statistics, 1990. Available at: http://www.healthyfridge.org/women_heart_disease.html. Accessed May 1, 2008.

[5] Robertson R. Women and cardiovascular disease: the risk of misperception and the need for action. Circulation 2001;103:2318–20.

[6] Christian A, Rosamond W, White A, et al. Nine-year trends and racial and ethnic disparities in women's awareness of heart disease and stroke: an American Heart Association National Study. J Womans Health (Larchmt) 2007;16(1):68–81.

[7] The heart truth. Available at: http://www.nhlbi.nih.gov/health/hearttruth/. Accessed November 7, 2007.

[8] American Heart Association go for red. Available at: www.goredforwomen.org. Accessed November 7, 2007.

[9] Mosca L, Appel L, Benjamin E, et al. Evidence-based guidelines for cardiovascular disease prevention in women. J Am Coll Cardiol 2004;43:900–21.

[10] Limacher M. Hormones and heart disease: what we thought, what we have learned, what we still need to know. Trans Am Clin Climatol Assoc 2002;113: 31–41.

[11] American College of Obstetrics and Gynecology Task Force for Hormone Therapy. Summary of balancing risks and benefits. Obstet Gynecol 2004; 104(4 Suppl):1S–129S.

[12] 2004 Surgeon General's report—the health consequences of smoking. Available at: http://www.cdc.gov/tobacco/data_statistics/sgr/sgr_2004/index.htm. Accessed November 7, 2007.

[13] Centers for Disease Control and Prevention. CDC United States national diabetes fact sheet. Available at: http://apps.nccd.cdc.gov/ddtstrs/FactSheet.aspx. Accessed November 7, 2007.

[14] Centers for Disease Control and Prevention. CDC Diabetes trend maps. Available at: http://www.cdc.gov/diabetes/statistics/maps/. Accessed November 7, 2007.

[15] The seventh report of the Joint National Committee on Prevention, Evaluation, and Treatment of High Blood Pressure (JNC 7, 2004). Available at: www.nhlbi.nih.gov/guidelines/hypertension/. Accessed November 7, 2007.

[16] American Heart Association. Third report of the NCEP Expert Panel on ATP III. Circulation 2002; 106:3143–421.

[17] Maron DJ. The epidemiology of low levels of high-density lipoprotein cholesterol in patients with and without coronary artery disease. Am J Cardiol 2000;86:11L–4L.

[18] Centers for Disease Control and Prevention. Obesity trend maps. Available at: http://www.cdc.gov/nccdphp/dnpa/obesity/trend/index.htm. Accessed November 7, 2007.

[19] US Department of Health and Human Services. Recommended dietary allowances. 2005. Available at: http://www.health.gov/dietaryguidelines/dga2005/document/default.htm. Accessed May 1, 2008.

[20] McDonald's USA nutrition facts. Available at: http://www.mcdonalds.com/app_controller.nutrition.index1.html. Accessed November 7, 2007.

[21] National Heart Lung and Blood Institute. Food portion distortion. Available at: http://hp2010.nhlbihin.net/portion/. Accessed November 7, 2007.

[22] US Food and Drug Administration. Questions and answers about *trans* fat nutrition labeling. Available at: http://www.cfsan.fda.gov/~dms/qatrans2.html#s5q3. Accessed November 7, 2007.

[23] Pate R, Pratt M, Blair S, et al. Physical activity and public health. JAMA 1995;273(5):402–7.

[24] Manson J, Hu F, Rich-Edwards J, et al. A prospective study of walking compared with vigorous exercise in the prevention of coronary heart disease in women. N Engl J Med 1999;341(9):650–8.

[25] American Heart Association. Choose to move. Available at: www.choosetomove.org. Accessed November 7, 2007.

[26] Rosenfeld A. State of the heart: building science to improve women's cardiovascular health. Am J Crit Care 2006;15(6):556–66.

[27] McSweeney J, Cody M, O'Sullivian P, et al. Women's early warning symptoms of acute myocardial infarction. Circulation 2003;108:2619–23.

[28] McSweeney J, Cody M, O'Sullivan P, et al. Black women's symptoms of coronary heart disease. AHA Scientific Sessions. Dallas (TX): American Heart Association; 2005.

[29] Wenger N. You've come a long way, baby. Cardiovascular health and disease in women, problems and prospects. Circulation 2004;109:558–60.

[30] Anderson J, Adams C, Antman E, et al. ACC/AHA 2007 guidelines for NSTEMI/UA. J Am Coll Cardiol 2007;50:1–57.

[31] Antman E, Anbe D, Armstrong P, et al. ACC/AHA guidelines for STEMI. J Am Coll Cardiol 2004; 44(3):E1–211.

[32] Lefler L, Bondy K. Women's delay in seeking treatment with myocardial infarction: a meta-synthesis. J Cardiovasc Nurs 2004;19(4):251–68.

[33] De Luca G, Suryapranata H, Ottervanger P, et al. Time delay to treatment and mortality in primary angioplasty for acute myocardial infarction. Circulation 2004;109:1223–5.

[34] Lee P, Alexander K, Hammill B, et al. Representation of elderly and women in published randomized trials of acute coronary syndrome. JAMA 2001; 286(6):708–13.

[35] Vaccarino V, Qiu Lin Z, Kasl S, et al. Sex differences in health after coronary artery bypass surgery. Circulation 2003;108:2642–7.

[36] Scott LB, Allen JK. Provider's perceptions of factors affecting women's referral to outpatient cardiac rehabilitation programs: an exploratory study. J Cardiopulm Rehabil 2004;24:387–91.

[37] Lansky A, Hochmann J, Ward P, et al. Percutaneous coronary intervention and adjunctive pharmacotherapy in women. Circulation 2005;111:940–53.

ELSEVIER
SAUNDERS

Crit Care Nurs Clin N Am 20 (2008) 265–271

CRITICAL CARE
NURSING CLINICS
OF NORTH AMERICA

Kawasaki Disease: A Ride for Little Girls Too!

Lynn Smith Schnautz, RN, MSN, CCRN, CCNS, NP-C[a,b,*],
Patricia Leggett, RN, BSN, CCRN, CMSRN[a]

[a]*Deaconess Hospital, Evansville, IN, USA*
[b]*Integrity Family Physicians, Evansville, IN, USA*

Addie's red dress

Addie, a 1-year-old white female, presents to the emergency room at a local hospital accompanied by her parents (Fig. 1). Her mother says her symptoms include inconsolable moaning, fever of 102°F and higher for 1 week unrelieved with alternating Motrin or Tylenol every 4 hours, strawberry-coated tongue, drooling with halitosis, decreased fluid intake (less than one bottle of whole milk in the past 24 hours), one wet diaper in the past 24 hours, 2+ edema of hands, slight edema of feet, and weight loss of 2 kg in 1 week. Her mother said her symptoms began 1 week ago with a fever of 102° unrelieved by alternating Tylenol and Motrin every 4 hours for 48 hours.

Addie was evaluated by the family practitioner after 2 days, who ordered a complete blood cell (CBC) count, which showed a white blood cell (WBC) count of 7000 cells/mm³ and a neutrophil count of 45,000 cells/mm³. The family practitioner believed the illness to be viral in nature and instructed the mother to continue to rotate Tylenol and Motrin every 4 hours, increase fluid intake, monitor diaper count, and call the office if Addie was not better in 2 days.

The fever was not relieved in 2 days and Addie had developed white vesicles on her tongue, accompanied by drooling and halitosis. Her fluid consumption had decreased to 4 ounces of whole milk every 8 hours. She had an erythematous fine flat rash noted on her trunk, which lasted less than

24 hours. She was evaluated by her family nurse practitioner, who ordered a repeat CBC.

Laboratory results showed a WBC count of 17,000 cells/mm³ with elevated bands and segs. The diagnosis was changed to bacterial infection and Augmentin was prescribed. She received one dose of Augmentin 8 hours before admission. According to her parents, she had taken Augmentin in the past for an ear infection and did not have a reaction. When her parents noticed the severe swelling in her hands, they brought her to the emergency room.

Initial assessment in the emergency room showed a 1-year-old white female who was inconsolable, moaning while being held by mother. She was drooling with halitosis and had flushed cheeks, 2+ edematous hands that resembled sausage rolls, and slight edema of feet bilaterally. Initial laboratory work showed normochromic, normocytic anemia, a WBC count of 19,600 cells/mm³, monocyte count of 15 cells/mm³, sedimentation rate of 93 mm/h, platelet count of 587 cells/mm³, sodium level of 134 mEq/L, and a chloride level of 99 mmol/L, with unremarkable urinalysis. She is admitted to the pediatric floor for observation and ordered fluids, Tylenol, and Motrin.

Her history shows a healthy 1-year-old, delivered at 41 weeks, with no complications at birth, one ear infection at 6 months, and otherwise healthy. She has two older sisters, neither of which is currently ill and both have been healthy since birth. She attends daycare 2 to 3 days per week and the parents report that no other children are ill at the facility. On further investigation, it was established that Addie had been exposed to carpet cleaner 14 days before symptoms developed.

* Corresponding author.
E-mail address: lynn_schnautz@deaconess.com (L.S. Schnautz).

0899-5885/08/$ - see front matter © 2008 Elsevier Inc. All rights reserved.
doi:10.1016/j.ccell.2008.03.013

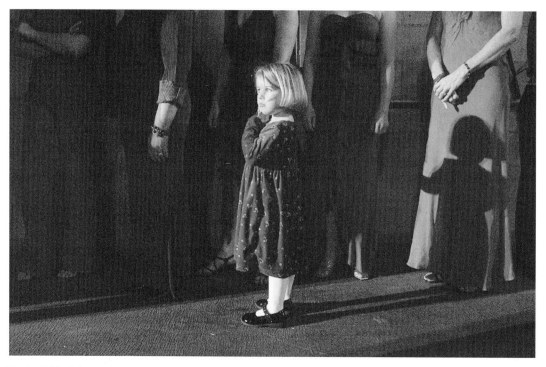

Fig. 1. Addie Schnautz, age 3 years, Evansville, Indiana. (*Courtesy of* Justin Rumbach, Evansville Courier Press, Evansville, Indiana).

Her pediatrician was called to evaluate her for Kawasaki disease, and a pediatric cardiologist was consulted. Addie was moved to the pediatric intensive care unit. Her initial EKG showed normal sinus tachycardia at a rate of 158 beats per minute. She was treated with IgG intravenously, fluids, and Tylenol/Motrin every 4 hours.

Kawasaki disease

Kawasaki disease or syndrome is an acute, self-limited, generalized vasculitis of unknown origin. First described in 1967 by Tomisaku Kawasaki, the disease was known as *mucocutaneous lymph node syndrome*. It is a distinctive clinical illness characterized by fever, redness of the eyes, diffuse red rash, redness and swelling of the hands and feet, and enlarged lymph nodes in the neck [1]. Coronary artery aneurysms or ectasia develop in approximately 15% to 25% of untreated children and may lead to ischemic heart disease or sudden death [2]. Kawasaki disease has replaced rheumatic fever as the leading cause of acquired heart disease in children in the United States and Japan [3].

Prevalence and incidence

Kawasaki disease has been reported throughout the world. In the United States, the disease has been increasingly recognized since the 1970s, and several regional outbreaks have been reported since 1976. Kawasaki disease occurs more often in boys than girls (approximately 1.5:1 ratio). Approximately 80% of affected children are younger than 5 years. Fewer than 2% of children experience recurrences [2].

The disease occurs year-round, but more cases are reported in the winter and spring. Annual incidence rates in the United States and Canada range from approximately 6 to 11 cases per 100,000 children younger than 5 years. As many as 3500 children in the United States are hospitalized each year because of Kawasaki disease. Although the absolute number of cases in the United States is greatest in white children, the incidence rates in North America are highest in children of Asian ethnicity, especially Japanese or Korean [4].

Literature from Japan best documents the rates of KD recurrence and familial occurrence. The recurrence rate of KD in Japan is reported to be approximately 3%. The proportion of cases with a positive family history is approximately 1%. Within 1 year after onset of the first case in a family, the rate in a sibling is 2.1%, which is a relative risk of approximately 10-fold compared with the unaffected Japanese population; approximately 50% of the second cases develop within 10 days of the first case.

The risk for occurrence in twins is approximately 13%. Higher rates of Kawasaki disease in siblings and twins suggest a possible role for genetic predisposition that interacts with exposure to the causative agent or agents in the environment. The reported occurrence of Kawasaki disease in children of parents who had the illness in childhood also supports the contribution of genetic factors [2].

Associations of Kawasaki disease with antecedent respiratory illness and exposure to carpet cleaning have been documented. Other factors associated with Kawasaki disease include preexisting eczema, humidifier use, and living near a standing body of water [5].

Pathophysiology

According to McCance and Huether [6], Kawasaki disease progresses pathologically and clinically in the following stages: (1) stage I, or acute phase (days 0–12), during which the small capillaries, arterioles, and venules become inflamed, as does the heart itself; (2) stage II, or subacute phase (days 12–25), during which the inflammation spreads to larger vessels and aneurysms of the coronary arteries develop; (3) stage III, or convalescent phase (days 26–40), during which the medium-size arteries begin the granulation process, causing coronary artery thickening; inflammation resolves in the microcirculation; and formation of thrombi increases; and (4) stage IV, or chronic phase (days 40 and beyond), during which the vessels develop scarring, intimal thickening, and calcification, and stenosis of coronary arteries develops.

Although the coronary arteries are virtually always involved in autopsy cases, Kawasaki disease is a generalized systemic vasculitis involving blood vessels throughout the body. Aneurysms may occur in other extraparenchymal muscular arteries, such as the celiac, mesenteric, femoral, iliac, renal, axillary, and brachial arteries.

The media of affected vessels show edematous dissociation of the smooth muscle cells, which is most obvious toward the exterior. Endothelial cells swelling and subendothelial edema are seen, but the internal elastic lamina remains intact. An influx of neutrophils is found in the early stages (7–9 days after onset), with a rapid transition to large mononuclear cells in concert with lymphocytes (predominately CD8+ T cells) and immunoglobulin A (IgA) plasma cells. Destruction of the internal elastic lamina and eventually fibroblastic proliferation occur at this stage. Matrix metalloproteinases are prominent in the remodeling process. Active inflammation is replaced over several weeks to months through progressive fibrosis, with scar formation [2].

Arterial remodeling or revascularization may occur in Kawasaki disease with coronary arteritis. Progressive stenosis in the disease results from active remodeling with intimal proliferation and neoangiogenesis; the intima is markedly thickened and consists of linearly arranged microvessels, a layer that is rich in smooth muscle cells, and fibrous layers. Several growth factors are prominently expressed at the inlet and outlet of aneurysms, where they are activated by high shear stress [2].

Pathologic findings in lymph nodes include thrombotic arteriolitis and severe lymphadenitis with necrosis. Lymph node biopsies performed in the first week of the illness show abnormal hyperplasia of reticular cells around the postcapillary venule [2].

Striking immune perturbations occur in acute Kawasaki disease, including marked cytokine cascade stimulation and endothelial cell activation. The key steps leading to coronary arteritis are still being clarified, but endothelial cell activation, CD68+ monocyte/macrophages, CD8+ (cytotoxic) lymphocytes, and oligoclonal IgA plasma cells seem to be involved. The prominence of IgA plasma cells in the respiratory tract, which is similar to findings in fatal viral respiratory infections, suggests a respiratory portal of entry of an etiologic agent or agents.

Enzymes, including matrix metalloproteinases that are capable of damaging arterial wall integrity, may be important in the development of aneurismal dilatation. Vascular endothelial growth factor (MCAF or MCP1), tumor necrosis factor α, and various interleukins also seem to play an important role in the vasculitis process [2].

The origin of Kawasaki disease remains unknown, although clinical and epidemiologic features strongly suggest an infectious cause. Efforts to identify an infectious agent in Kawasaki disease using conventional bacterial and viral cultures, serologic methods, and animal inoculation, have failed to identify an infectious cause [2].

An attractive hypothesis is that Kawasaki disease is caused by a ubiquitous infectious agent that produces clinically apparent disease only in certain genetically predisposed individuals, particularly Asians. Its rarity in the first few months of life and in adults suggests an agent to which the latter are immune and from which young infants are protected by passive maternal antibodies. Because little evidence exists of person-to-person transmission, this hypothesis assumes that most infected children experience asymptomatic infection with only a small fraction developing overt clinical features of Kawasaki disease [2].

The hypothesis that Kawasaki disease is related to a bacterial superantigenic toxin has been suggested because of the reported selective expansion of VB2 and VB8 T-cell receptor families, but this theory remains controversial. Other investigators support an alternative hypothesis that the immune response in Kawasaki disease is oligoclonal (antigen-driven) rather than polyclonal (superantigen-driven), and IgA plasma cells play a central role [2].

The possibility also exists that Kawasaki disease results from an immunologic response that is triggered by any of several different microbial agents. Support for this hypothesis includes documented infection from different microorganisms in different individual cases, failure to detect a single microbiological or environmental agent after almost 3 decades of study, and analogies to other syndromes caused by multiple agents. This hypothesis is somewhat difficult to reconcile with the distinctive clinical/laboratory picture of Kawasaki disease with its epidemiologic features [2].

Clinical features

During the acute stage of Kawasaki disease, children will display an elevated temperature (usually $>104°$ F) that does not respond to Tylenol, Motrin, or antibiotics. Children will be extremely irritable disproportionate to the degree of fever. Bilateral conjunctivitis is noted but not associated with exudate. Changes in lips and the oral cavity may include pharyngeal edema, dry/fissured or swollen lips [7], and strawberry tongue [8]. Changes in extremities may include erythema [7] and edema, which may limit movement and cause children to refuse to bear weight. Children

may display polymorphous rash [7] and cervical lymphadenopathy. Hepatic dysfunction may also develop. Cardiac complications that may develop include myocarditis and pericarditis [9].

The subacute stage is characterized by persistent irritability and anorexia. Usually the fever has resolved by this stage, but if it persists the outcome is less favorable due to the greater risk of cardiac complications. Thrombosis develops and the platelet count may be greater than 1 million. Desquamation of the fingertips and toes begins at this time. Aneurysm formation may also occur during this stage [9].

The most significant clinical finding that persists during the convalescent stage is the presence of coronary artery aneurysms. The development of coronary aneurysms is the main feature of the chronic stage of Kawasaki disease. The cardiac complications will endure a lifetime of significance because the aneurysms formed in childhood may rupture in adulthood [9]. Noncardiac manifestations of Kawasaki disease are shown in Box 1 [10].

Because no specific laboratory test exists for diagnosing Kawasaki disease in children, diagnosis is based on signs and symptoms. Children must exhibit five of the following criteria to be diagnosed with Kawasaki disease: (1) fever for five or more days; (2) bilateral conjunctival infection without exudation; (3) changes in the oral mucous membranes (ie, erythema, dryness, fissuring of the lips, oropharyngeal reddening, strawberry tongue); (4) changes in the extremities (ie, peripheral edema, peripheral erythema, desquamation of palms and soles) [9], particularly periungual peeling; (5) polymorphous rash, often accentuated in the perineal area; or (6) lymphadenopathy [6].

Significant laboratory findings are identified during the various stages of Kawasaki disease. A mild-to-moderate normochromic anemia is observed in the acute stage, along with a moderate to alarmingly elevated WBC count with a shift to the left. Erythrocyte sedimentation rate, C-reactive protein, and serum alpha-1 antitrypsin are also elevated during this phase. During the subacute stage, platelet count elevation is the outstanding marker. Platelet levels as high as 2 million have been documented in the literature [9]. During the convalescent stage, the levels of platelets and other markers begin to return to baseline. Laboratory values may require 6 to 8 weeks to normalize.

An ECG may identify the presence of various conduction abnormalities or the presence of any

Box 1. Noncardiac manifestations of Kawasaki disease: associated signs and symptoms

Gastrointestinal
Vomiting
Diarrhea
Gallbladder hydrops
Elevated transaminases

Blood
Acute phase
  Elevated erythrocyte sedimentation
    rate or creatinine phosphokinase
  Leukocytosis
  Hypoalbuminemia
  Mild anemia
Subacute phase
  Thrombocytosis (usually second
    to third week of illness)

Renal
Sterile pyuria
Proteinuria
Respiratory
Cough
Rhinorrhea
Infiltrate on chest radiograph

Joint
Arthralgia
Arthritis

Neurology
Mononuclear pleocytosis
  of cerebrospinal fluid
Irritability
Facial palsy

From Hay WW, Levin MJ, Sondheimer JM, et al. Current pediatric diagnosis and treatment in pediatrics. 17th edition. New York: Lange Medical Books/McGraw-Hill; 2005. p. 602–3; with permission.

ischemic changes. Children who have Kawasaki disease are at risk for developing a myocardial infarction. An echocardiogram is the preferred study to identify coronary aneurysms during the acute stage of Kawasaki disease. A chest radiograph should be performed to assess baseline findings and confirm any suspicions of congestive heart failure [9].

Collaborative care

Advanced practice nurses (APNs) must have extremely astute assessment skills to diagnose children who have Kawasaki disease. APNs are typically the health care providers children see in the family practice office or clinic, when the first signs of Kawasaki disease may present. APNs must collaborate and discuss these suspicious signs and symptoms with the family practitioner.

Because diagnosis is based on the child presenting with a fever lasting at least 5 days, explicit instructions must be given to parents or legal guardians about the need to seek additional medical attention if the fever is of less duration when first examined.

Children who have Kawasaki disease should be admitted to the hospital through the emergency room, or directly to the pediatric intensive care unit if diagnosed in the office. The APN should collaborate with the attending physician to help direct care. A consultation should be obtained with a pediatric cardiologist, and possible transfer to a tertiary pediatric facility may be necessary.

A multidisciplinary approach to treatment should be initiated and include members from nursing, pharmacy, physicians (ie, pediatric attending, pediatric cardiologist, and perhaps pediatric cardiothoracic surgeon), laboratory, echocardiogram technology, case management, physical therapy, nutrition, and clergy. The emergency room and pediatric intensive care nurses provide children and parents with physical, emotional, and spiritual care, and play a key role in coordinating the care among the multiple members of the health care team. The nurses will also be responsible for teaching parents about Kawasaki disease and including them in the patient plan of care.

Baseline intravenous access, cardiac monitoring, laboratory tests, and cardiac workup should be completed. APNs should also rule out the possibility of sepsis or meningitis. The initial medical management of Kawasaki disease involves the use of gamma globulin and aspirin as anti-inflammatory agents and long-term anticoagulation. Consultation with the pharmacy staff may help determine the proper dose and potential side effects of these medications.

Gammagard (IVIG), an immune globulin, is administered at 400 mg/kg per day intravenously in a single daily infusion for 4 days or single dose of 2 g/kg intravenously infused over 12 hours. Aspirin inhibits prostaglandin synthesis, which prevents the formation of platelet-aggregating thromboxane A2, and is administered in combination with the gamma globulin. The dosage is 80 to 100 mg/kg per day orally divided four times daily for 2 weeks initially, then 3 to 5 mg/kg orally every day for 6 to 8 weeks maintenance [11]. Children who have coronary artery aneurysms will receive aspirin for prolonged periods under the direction of the pediatric cardiologist.

Children for whom the initial IVIG failed will receive a second dose at a rate of 2 g/kg intravenously, accompanied by the use of corticosteroids. The most commonly used steroid regimen is intravenous methylprednisolone at 30 mg/kg for 2 to 3 hours, administered once daily for 1 to 3 days. Other treatment options plasma exchange, abciximab, and cytotoxic agents such as cyclophosphamide [2].

Treatment of coronary thrombosis may require the use of aspirin, low molecular weight heparin, warfarin, streptokinase, abciximab, dipyridamole, or dipyridamole therapy. Children who have Kawasaki disease may require interventional cardiac catheterization techniques, such as balloon angioplasty, rotational ablation, and stent placement. Coronary bypass graft procedures may be necessary because of ischemia from myocardial infarction. A small number of patients who have Kawasaki disease have undergone cardiac transplantation for severe myocardial dysfunction, ventricular arrhythmias, and coronary arterial lesions [2].

Repeat laboratory values must be obtained in 6 to 8 weeks. An echocardiogram should be repeated in the second or third week, and again at 1 month after all other laboratory results have returned to normal (usually 6–8 weeks). Pediatric cardiologists determine how often to repeat an echocardiogram based on the development of any aneurysms. Table 1 reviews the risk stratification and recommended follow-up [10].

The Web site of the Kawasaki Disease Foundation (http://www.kdfoundation.org) provides additional resources and support for the family.

Addie's red dress: conclusion

Addie was treated with one dose of IVIG and started on 200 mg of aspirin four times daily. Her fever broke within 24 hours of receiving IVIG; she was alert, oriented, and running around her hospital room. Her echocardiogram was unremarkable and she was discharged on 200 mg of aspirin four times daily for 6 weeks. Her repeat echocardiogram at 6 weeks and 1 year both were unremarkable. Today she is a vibrant 7-year-old in the first grade who enjoys swimming. She is leading a heart-healthy lifestyle, with proper diet and exercise. She is a spokesperson for Kawasaki disease and has participated in her local American Heart Association's Go Red Campaign for the past 2 years.

Table 1
Long-term management of Kawasaki disease

Risk level	Definition	Management guidelines
I	No coronary artery changes at any stage of the illness	No acetyl salicylic acid (ASA) is needed beyond the subacute phase (6–8 weeks) No follow-up beyond the first year
II	Transient ectasia of coronary arteries during the acute phase	Same as level I, or clinical follow-up plus ECG every 3–5 years
III	Single small to medium coronary aneurysm	ASA until abnormality resolves Annual follow-up with ECG and echocardiogram if younger than 10 years, and every other year stress testing if older than 10 years
IV	Giant aneurysm or multiple small to medium aneurysms without obstruction	Long-term ASA or warfarin Annual follow-up with ECG, echo, and stress testing (in those older than 20 years)
V	Coronary artery obstruction	Long-term ASA or warfarin or calcium channel blocker to reduce myocardial oxygen consumption Echocardiogram and ECG every 6 months Stress testing and Holter examination annually

From Hay WW, Levin MJ, Sondheimer JM, et al. Current pediatric diagnosis and treatment in pediatrics. 17th edition. New York: Lange Medical Books/McGraw-Hill; 2005. p. 603; with permission.

Summary

Kawasaki disease is the leading cause of acquired heart disease in children in the United States. Its prevalence is highest among boys of Japanese or Korean heritage, but it also occurs in girls. Although the exact origin of the disease is unknown, clinical and epidemiologic features strongly suggest an infectious cause. The disease does not have one specific diagnostic test, and therefore diagnosis is based on the clinical presentation. A multidisciplinary team approach to the care of patients who have Kawasaki disease is fundamental. Critical care, emergency room, and advanced practice nurses are instrumental in the diagnosis and treatment of Kawasaki disease.

Acknowledgment

The authors would like to thank Karen Barnes-Ellis, RN, MSN, NP-C, and Drs. James Jenison, Chip Walsh, and David Atkinson for their excellent clinical assessment skills and early recognition of Kawasaki disease. Many thanks to Dr. Newburger and colleagues for their pioneering spirit in educating health care providers about Kawasaki disease.

References

[1] American Heart Association (2007, Fall). Kawasaki disease. Available at: http://www.americanheart.org/presenter.jhtml?identifier=4634. Accessed November 27, 2007.

[2] Newburger JW, Takahashi M, Gerber MA, et al. Diagnosis, treatment, and long-term management of Kawasaki disease: a statement for health professionals from the Committee on Rheumatic Fever, Endocarditis and Kawasaki Disease, Council on Cardiovascular Disease in the Young, America Heart Association. Circulation 2004;110:2747–71.

[3] Hempel K. Kawasaki disease. 2002. Available at: http://www.tfn.net/HealthGazette/kawasaki.html. Accessed November 27, 2007.

[4] American Academy of Family Physicians. Taubert KA, Shulman ST. Cardiovascular medicine: Kawasaki disease. Available at: http://www.aafp.org/afp/990600ap/3093.html. Accessed November 27, 2007.

[5] Lehman TJ. A common manifestation of an uncommon agent, or an uncommon manifestation of a common agent? 2002. Available at: http://www.goldscout.com/kdmike1.html. Accessed November 27, 2007.

[6] McCance KL, Huether SE. Pathophysiology: the biologic basis for disease in adults and children. 4th edition. St. Louis (MO): Mosby; 2002. p. 1075–6.

[7] Habif TP, Campbell JL, Chapman MS, et al. Skin disease: diagnosis and treatment. 2nd edition. Philadelphia: Elsevier; 2005. p. 270–3.

[8] Seidel HM, Ball JW, Dains JE, et al. Mosby's guide to physical examination. 6th edition. St. Louis (MO): Mosby; 2006. p. 490.

[9] Parrillo S, Parrillo C. Pediatrics, Kawasaki disease. emedicine from webmd 2001;2(12):1–10. Available at: http://www.emedicine.com/emerg/topic811.htm. Accessed November 27, 2007.

[10] Hay WW, Levin MJ, Sondheimer JM, et al. Current pediatric diagnosis & treatment. 17th edition. New York: Lange Medical Books/McGraw-Hill; 2005. p. 602–3.

[11] Micromedex. Kawasaki disease. Micromedex (R) healthcare series: diseasedex clinical points emergency medicine, 126. 2007. Available at: http://www.drugs.com/enc/kawasaki-disease.html. Accessed November 27, 2007.

ELSEVIER
SAUNDERS

Crit Care Nurs Clin N Am 20 (2008) 273–276

CRITICAL CARE
NURSING CLINICS
OF NORTH AMERICA

Acute Coronary Syndromes and Women: There are Differences

Eugenia Welch, BSN, RN, CCRN[a],*,
Damon B. Cottrell, MS, RN, CCNS, CCRN, CNS-BC, CEN[b]

[a]Emergency Department, Presbyterian Hospital of Kaufman, 850 Highway 243 West,
Kaufman, TX 75142, USA
[b]Cardiology, Washington Hospital Center, 110 Irving Street, NW, 4NE-4082, Washington, DC 20010, USA

Cardiovascular disease is the leading cause of death for men and women in the United States [1–3]. Today, more women in the United States die from heart disease than from breast, ovarian, and uterine cancer combined, and myocardial infarction is the leading cause of death from heart disease [4,5]. Women who survive an acute myocardial infarction (AMI) have an increased risk of suffering another or of developing heart failure [5]. A number of therapies are available to treat AMI and can be effective in reducing mortality and morbidity; maximum benefit, however, occurs with rapidly initiated treatment. Unfortunately, many individuals wait several hours and in some cases even days before seeking treatment.

Acute coronary syndrome (ACS) is an important aspect of heart disease for clinicians to consider in women. "ACS" is a broad term used to describe a continuum of disorders that consists of unstable angina, non–ST-elevation myocardial infarction (NSTEMI), and ST-elevation myocardial infarction (STEMI). In this article, the term "ACS" is used to refer to unstable angina, NSTEMI, and STEMI. These manifestations share pathophysiologic mechanisms that require rapid assessment, diagnosis, and treatment to achieve optimal treatment and outcomes [6].

Historically, women were excluded from research investigations to protect them from any ill effects of clinical research [1]. Perhaps for this reason, coronary heart disease is "underdiagnosed,

undertreated, and under-researched" in women [3], and the body of evidence seems to point towards three explanations: sex-based physiology, provider bias, and psychosocial influences [3]. Women account for only 20% to 30% of participants in clinical trials [3]. Fortunately, as research evolves more is being learned about gender-specific aspects of care.

Anatomic differences

Women have a higher incidence of vascular abnormalities (eg, Reynaud's phenomenon, migraine headaches, and vasospastic disorders) than men [7]. Women characteristically have smaller and less compliant arteries than men [7]. Gender differences in outcomes previously were attributed to small vessel size in women, although few studies included the size and quality of the vessels in the analyses of results [8]. In the study completed by Mickleborough and colleagues [8], researchers found that despite smaller body size, the women were no more likely than men to have a grafted vessel smaller than 1.5 mm. Because the coronary arteries in women typically are smaller than those in men, they often are more difficult to revascularize [9].

There also is evidence suggesting that sex hormones play a role in the pathophysiology of vascular disease [7]. Before menopause, women are protected from cardiovascular diseases when compared with men [10]. This protection has been attributed to the protective effects of the female hormones such as estrogen [10]. ACS occurs later in women, and this delay generally is believed to result from the protective influences of

* Corresponding author.
E-mail address: ecwelch6@sbcglobal.net (E. Welch).

0899-5885/08/$ - see front matter © 2008 Elsevier Inc. All rights reserved.
doi:10.1016/j.ccell.2008.03.006

ccnursing.theclinics.com

the reproductive hormone estrogen [11]. As estrogen levels decline during and after menopause, the cardiovascular risk for women increases. Because of this belief, it was assumed that hormone replacement therapy would decrease the risk of cardiovascular disease in postmenopausal women. Research, however, has demonstrated that hormone replacement therapy in postmenopausal women is not cardioprotective [12,13].

Symptoms

Women typically are older than men at the diagnosis of ACS, have more comorbidities such as diabetes mellitus and hypertension, and are less likely to be smokers [9,14–16]. Differences in outcomes between men and women may occur because women have more comorbid conditions, smaller body size, and generally are older at the time of the event [3]. Women typically are 10 or more years older than their male counterparts when they experience a first cardiac event [9,15,16].

Recent studies have indicated that women suffering from AMIs present differently than men. Women are less likely to present with chest pain as the chief complaint and are more likely to present with transient pain in addition to pain described as "sharp" or "stabbing" [8,15]. Women report more nausea and/or vomiting and are more likely to present with dyspnea, referred back and neck pain, indigestion, and palpitations [2,4,6,9,14,15]. Women also are less likely to report diaphoresis [15]. These correlations may be age related, because atypical presentation of an AMI is more common in older patients [15].

Patients presenting without chest pain tend to be older than those presenting with typical symptoms. These patients are more likely to be women, are more likely to have a history of hypertension, diabetes, or heart failure, and are less likely to have a history of smoking, hyperlipidemia, or percutaneous intervention [17]. Patients who present with atypical symptoms also take longer to present to the hospital [17]. Women have been reported to take longer seeking medical treatment, and this delay may explain their increased risk of poor outcomes [2].

Treatment delay

There are reports of delay in seeking treatment by women, although these reports are not necessarily current [18–21]. Rosenfeld and colleagues [5] reported more recent studies that indicated similar findings of delay in women and completed a qualitative study of 52 women in an attempt to understand the rationale for this delay. These investigators also categorized patients seeking treatment as (1) those who know they need treatment and seek it, (2) those who know they need treatment and let another person take charge, (3) those who know they need treatment and seek it on their own terms, (4) those who manage an alternative hypothesis, and (5) those who minimize the symptoms. Still, this concept that women delay seeking treatment seems to be somewhat uncertain, because other studies have found that there is no difference between genders in delayed treatment seeking or that such delay has no statistical significance [2,22].

Differences in treatment

ACS and AMI have poor outcomes in women. Although the outcomes originally were thought to result from physicians' gender bias, more evidence points toward the later onset of cardiac disease, the higher incidence of comorbid conditions and risk factors, and a lower functional status in women [7]. There also is speculation that these poor outcomes may be associated with later diagnosis and suboptimal care [3].

It seems that women receive less aggressive treatment than men, including underuse of revascularization procedures [7,9,16,23,24]. Although this difference is identified in the literature, women also tend to have more urgent procedures, rather than routine procedures; this tendency has been attributed to delay in seeking treatment [9].

Women suspected of having heart disease were less likely than men to receive indicated diagnostic tests and procedures [3], including coronary angiography and other appropriate noninvasive studies such as stress testing [24]. In a study completed by Martinez-Selles and colleagues [24] in 2005, the data demonstrated that women had fewer noninvasive studies and angiographies than men and that this gap worsened in patients aged 75 years and older.

Women who have ACS, especially those who have NSTEMI, have a higher percentage of normal coronary arteries as visualized on angiogram than do men; however, they tend to have worse outcomes [6,16,25]. This paradox can make diagnosis and treatment a greater challenge in women. This disease seems to be less common in women but more deadly [16].

For reasons that are poorly understood, women tend to have higher rates of complications associated with bleeding than men [9,16]. Gender differences also have been seen in glycoprotein IIb/IIIa use in women, with increased rates of myocardial infarction and deaths [16]. In 2006 Daly and colleagues [23] completed a study of 3779 patients to examine the impact of gender on the management of stable angina. The researchers reported antiplatelet therapy was used significantly less often in women at initial assessment and at 1 year [23]. Other differences in pharmacologic treatment included a significantly lower use of lipid-lowering therapy in women [23].

In 2006 Gold and Krumholz [15] used data from the Cooperative Cardiovascular Project and National Heart Failure Project to examine gender differences in the treatment of acute myocardial infarction and heart failure. Their results were somewhat different from those of previous notions. They found gender was not a factor in the use of beta-blockers and fibrinolytic therapy, but they did report a slightly lower use of aspirin by women at admission and at discharge.

Tako-tsubo cardiomyopathy

Tako-tsubo cardiomyopathy also has been referred to in the literature as "apical ballooning syndrome," "stress-induced cardiomyopathy," and "broken heart syndrome." The term "tako-tsubo syndrome" is used because the syndrome originally was described in the Japanese population, and on ventriculogram the syndrome was characterized by an apical ballooning shaped like the bowl ("tsubo") used to catch octopus ("tako") [26,27]. Tako-tsubo cardiomyopathy primarily affects postmenopausal women [28–30]. The electrocardiogram changes in tako-tsubo syndrome are similar to those in STEMI [26,27,31], and it is quite difficult to differentiate between these two syndromes. A key distinguishing element, however, is the absence of coronary artery disease. The clinical features that may be somewhat different from those of STEMI include chest pain at rest or dyspnea alone, and there are rare reports of syncope [27]. Other clinical findings may include a hemodynamically stable patient, hypotension, and symptoms consistent with mild or moderate heart failure [27]. Treatment of tako-tsubo syndrome should follow that of AMI until AMI is ruled out. The prognosis is generally good, especially in patients who do not have comorbid disease [27].

Psychosocial implications

It has been reported that women minimize symptoms and fail to view themselves as being at risk for ACS [11,32]. The tendency to minimize the impact of the disease has been suggested as a rationale for the reported delay in seeking treatment [11,33]. This finding, which has been validated by other studies, points to the importance of educating patients and the public.

Coping strategies are another consideration in caring for women who have ACS. Qualitative research has demonstrated that women have a variety of coping strategies. It has been reported that meeting their household responsibilities are important to women and that, in general, women did not want to burden others with their health issues [11]. It also is significant that women report having less social support than men, even as long as 1 year after a first cardiac event [11].

Women who have ACS tend to be older, to have lower incomes, are more likely to be unmarried or widowed, and have a higher rate of anxiety and depression than men [11,14]. Depression may be as much as three times more common in women than in men [14]. These findings indicate a great need for psychosocial assessment and intervention.

Summary

As research that will shed light into gender-specific treatment of women who have ACS continues, knowledge will be gained, and it is hoped that patient outcomes will improve. The physiologic differences and differences in symptom reporting continue to be challenging, requiring practitioners to make critical decisions in treatment, including decisions regarding procedural diagnosis and pharmacologic therapy. With the known psychosocial aspects specific to women that may explain treatment delay, practitioners need to take every opportunity to educate their patients and the public about coronary artery disease, ACS, and AMI.

References

[1] Blauwet L, Hayes S, McManus D, et al. Low rate of sex-specific result reporting in cardiovascular trials. Mayo Clin Proc 2007;82:166–70.

[2] King K, McGuire M. Symptom presentation and time to seek care in women and men with acute myocardial infarction. Heart Lung 2007; 36:235–43.

[3] Rosenfeld A. State of the heart: building science to improve women's cardiovascular health. Am J Crit Care 2006;15:556–66.

[4] Patel H, Rosengren A, Ekman I. Symptoms in acute coronary syndromes: does sex make a difference? Am Heart J 2004;148:27–33.

[5] Rosenfeld AG, Lindauer A, Darney BG. Understanding treatment-seeking delay in women with acute myocardial infarction: descriptions of decision-making patterns. Am J Crit Care 2005;14: 285–93.

[6] Chen W, Woods S, Wilkie D, et al. Gender differences in symptom experiences of patients with acute coronary syndromes. J Pain Symptom Manage 2005;30:553–62.

[7] Anderson R, Pepine C. Gender differences in the treatment for acute myocardial infarction: bias or biology? Circulation 2007;115:823–6.

[8] Mickleborough L, Carson S, Ivanov J. Gender differences in quality of distal vessels: effect on results of coronary artery bypass grafting. J Thorac Cardiovasc Surg 2003;126:950–8.

[9] Mikhail G. Coronary revascularisation in women. Heart 2006;92(Suppl 3):iii19–23.

[10] Czubryt MP, Espira L, Lamoureux L, et al. The role of sex in cardiac function and disease. Can J Physiol Pharmacol 2006;84:93–109.

[11] Kristofferzon M, Lofmark R, Carlsson M. Myocardial infarction: gender differences in coping and social support. J Adv Nurs 2003;44:360–74.

[12] Mikkola TS, Clarkson TB. Coronary heart disease and postmenopausal hormone therapy: conundrum explained by timing? J Womens Health (Larchmt) 2006;15:51–3.

[13] Nicholson C. Cardiovascular disease in women. Nurs Stand 2007;21:43–7.

[14] DeVon H, Ryan C, Ochs A, et al. Symptoms across the continuum of acute coronary syndromes: differences between women and men. Am J Crit Care 2008;17:14–25.

[15] Gold L, Krumholz H. Gender differences in treatment of heart failure and acute myocardial infarction: a question of quality or epidemiology? Cardiol Rev 2006;14:180–6.

[16] Redberg R. Gender differences in acute coronary syndrome: invasive versus conservative approach. Cardiol Rev 2006;14:299–302.

[17] Brieger D, Eagle KA, Goodman SG, et al. Acute coronary syndromes without chest pain, an underdiagnosed and undertreated high-risk group: insights from the Global Registry of Acute Coronary Events. Chest 2004;126:461–9.

[18] Alonzo AA. The impact of the family and lay others on care-seeking during life-threatening episodes of suspected coronary artery disease. Soc Sci Med 1986;22:1297–311.

[19] Meischke H, Eisenberg MS, Larsen MP. Prehospital delay interval for patients who use emergency medical services: the effect of heart-related medical conditions and demographic variables. Ann Emerg Med 1993;22:1597–601.

[20] Turi ZG, Stone PH, Muller JE, et al. Implications for acute intervention related to time of hospital arrival in acute myocardial infarction. Am J Cardiol 1986;58:203–9.

[21] Zerwic J. Patient delay in seeking treatment for acute myocardial infarction symptoms. J Cardiovasc Nurs 1999;13:21–32.

[22] Meischke H, Larsen M, Eisenberg M. Gender differences in reported symptoms for acute myocardial infarction: impact on prehospital delay time interval. Am J Emerg Med 1998;16:363–6.

[23] Daly C, Clemens F, Lopez-Sendon J, et al. Gender differences in the management and clinical outcome of stable angina. Circulation 2006;113:490–8.

[24] Martinez-Selles M, Lopez-Palop R, Perez-David E, et al. Influence of age on gender differences in the management of acute inferior or posterior myocardial infarction. Chest 2005;128:792–7.

[25] Lagerqvist B, Safstrom K, Stahle E, et al. Is early invasive treatment of unstable coronary artery disease equally effective for both women and men? J Am Coll Cardiol 2001;38:41–8.

[26] Buchholz S, Rudan G. Tako-tsubo syndrome on the rise: a review of the current literature. Postgrad Med J 2007;83:261–4.

[27] Prasad A. Apical ballooning syndrome: an important differential diagnosis of acute myocardial infarction. Circulation 2007;115:e56–9.

[28] Akashi YJ, Nakazawa K, Sakakibara M, et al. The clinical features of takotsubo cardiomyopathy. QJM 2003;96:563–73.

[29] Inoue M, Shimizu M, Ino H, et al. Differentiation between patients with takotsubo cardiomyopathy and those with anterior acute myocardial infarction. Circ J 2005;69:89–94.

[30] Kurisu S, Sato H, Kawagoe T, et al. Tako-tsubo-like left ventricular dysfunction with ST-segment elevation: a novel cardiac syndrome mimicking acute myocardial infarction. Am Heart J 2002;143:448–55.

[31] Iqbal M, Moon J, Guttmann O, et al. Stress, emotion and the heart: tako-tsubo cardiomyopathy. Postgrad Med J 2006;82:e29.

[32] Worrall-Carter L, Jones T, Driscoll A. The experiences and adjustments of women following their first acute myocardial infarction. Contemp Nurse 2005; 19:211–21.

[33] Kentsch M, Rodemerk U, Muller-Esch G, et al. Emotional attitudes toward symptoms and inadequate coping strategies are major determinants of patient delay in acute myocardial infarction. Z Kardiol 2002;91:147–55.

ELSEVIER
SAUNDERS

Crit Care Nurs Clin N Am 20 (2008) 277–285

CRITICAL CARE
NURSING CLINICS
OF NORTH AMERICA

Cardiovascular Risk Assessment and Hyperlipidemia

Jerry Becker, MD, FACCP

The Heart Group, 415 West Columbia Street, Evansville, IN 47710, USA

This article reviews how to identify and risk-stratify patients at risk for developing coronary artery disease (CAD) or who already have CAD (or coronary risk equivalents), and how to manage their lipids. This discussion is directed toward the nurse, nurse practitioner, or physician assistant, who can and should play a pivotal role in identifying these patients and assisting the supervising physicians in management. In an April 8, 2004, editorial in the *New England Journal of Medicine*, Dr. Eric Topol wrote, "In the management of the atherosclerotic heart disease, statin drugs have already surpassed all other classes of medicines in reducing the incidence of the major adverse outcomes of death, heart attack and stroke" [1]. This statement compels physicians to identify, appropriately treat, and manage patients who can benefit from these medicines.

Risk for coronary artery disease

Within the next year, approximately 700,000 people in the United States will have a new coronary event and 500,000 will have a recurrent attack. In 2002, coronary disease caused one in five deaths [1,2]. Most clinical trials of statins show approximately a 30% relative risk reduction for coronary events when compared with placebo. Relative risk for all-cause mortality was reduced 30% in the Scandinavian Simvastatin Survival Study (4S), 22% in the Long-term Intervention with Pravastatin in Ischemic Disease (LIPID), and 13% in the Heart Protection Study (HPS) [2].

A brief review of evidence to treat

Before 1987 and the approval of lovastatin, the first 3-hydroxy-3-methlglutaryl coenzyme

E-mail address: beckercrc@aol.com

a reductase inhibitor (ie, statin), pharmacologic treatment consisted of resins, short-acting niacin, and fibrates. Clinical trials were generally small (a few hundred patients), but most showed that decrease in cholesterol was associated with a decrease in vascular events.

During the 1990s, the U.S. Food and Drug Administration (FDA) approved five additional statins, pravastatin, simvastatin, fluvastatin, and cerivastatin. Rosuvastatin, the last of the currently available statins, was approved in 2003. All are currently available for prescription except cerivastatin, which was removed from the market because it had greater side effects than the other available statins and showed no increased benefit. Over the next 15 years, numerous trials were reported, some with enrollments greater than 20,000 patients (HPS) [3].

The first landmark trial was the 4S trial, reported in 1994. This trial enrolled 4444 patients who had known coronary artery disease (CAD) and high cholesterol (212–309 mg/dL). Patients were randomized to either placebo or simvastatin, 20 to 40 mg, to achieve a cholesterol level of less than 200 mg/dL. After 5.4 years, 12% of patients died in the placebo group compared with 8% in the simvastatin group. It was calculated that 159 patients would need to be treated for 1 year to prevent one major event or death, or 30 patients over 5.4 years [4].

From 1994 to 2002 numerous trials were performed, both primary (without known disease) and secondary (known disease). Generally, a 30% relative reduction was seen [5].

The largest study is HPS, which randomized 20,536 patients who had some manifestation of CAD, cerebral vascular disease, peripheral vascular disease, type 1 or type 2 diabetes, or hypertension to receive either simvastatin, 40 mg daily,

doi:10.1016/j.ccell.2008.03.014

or placebo. All patients had cholesterol levels higher than 135 mg/dL, with no upper limits.

At the end of the 5-year trial, 12.9% patients died in the simvastatin group compared with 14.7% in the placebo group. Therefore, 55 patients would need to be treated for 5 years to prevent one death. The study population could be divided into three tertiles: those whose low-density lipoprotein cholesterol (LDL-C) is less than 115 mg/dL; those whose LDL-C is between 116 mg/dL and 135 mg/dL; and those whose LDL-C is greater than 135 mg/dL. Those who had LDL-C less than 115 mg/dL received just as much benefit as those who had LDL-C greater than 135 mg/dL. Those who had a 40 mg/dL reduction (despite LDL-C levels <100 mg/dL) received similar benefits. This large study strongly suggests that all high-risk patients, unless contraindicated, should be treated until they achieve a reduction of at least 40 mg/dL in LDL-C [3,6,7].

Standard coronary angiography visualizes the lumen of the coronary artery, and in many respects has been the gold standard for the presence or absence of CAD. However, it does not describe what occurs outside the luminal wall. Angiographers commonly find several 20% to 30% nonobstructive coronary lesions at catheterization of minimal CAD. Previously, these lesions were largely ignored and the prognosis was believed to be favorable.

Since the advent of coronary intravascular ultrasound (IVUS), these innocuous-appearing angiographic lesions have been recognized as being merely be the "tip of the iceberg." IVUS consists of advancing a small ultrasound catheter down the coronary artery. Ultrasound images can be sampled along the length of the artery. This technique provides an image of the vessel wall and the surrounding tissue beyond the wall. A motor-driven retractor that withdraws the IVUS catheter provides images at a 0.5-mm interval, supplying a cross-sectional image over a length of coronary artery. Using this information, the atheromatous burden can be calculated. More than 50% of acute myocardial infarctions are estimated to occur from coronary lesions in the range of 30%, strongly suggesting that these lesions that have not yet impinged on the coronary lumen are far from benign.

IVUS enables a baseline study to be performed, the patient to be treated with a statin, and then the study repeated to measure any changes that occur in the atheromatous burden. Two studies have been completed; the REVERSAL (Reversal of Atherosclerosis with Aggressive Lipid Lowering) trial in 2004 used IVUS to measure the progression, stabilization, or regression of coronary atheroma, and compared aggressive LDL-C lowering using atorvastatin, 80 mg, with a modest lowering using pravastatin, 40 mg. The aggressive LDL-C lowering was superior to modest lowering [8].

Another IVUS trial reported in 2006, ASTEROID (A Study to Evaluate the Effect of Rosuvastatin on Intravascular Ultrasound-Derived Coronary Atheroma Burden), used 40 mg of rosuvastatin to achieve LDL-C levels of 61 mg/dL. The IVUS method of measuring atheroma showed regression in 77.9% of patients and a strong linear relationship between the LDL-C achieved and the course of atherosclerosis [9–12].

Although the IVUS studies are impressive, clinical trials are needed to confirm whether lowering the levels below 70 mg /dL will translate into reduced vascular events.

Who to treat and how aggressively

In addition to a fasting lipid profile, two tools will be needed to assess patients: a risk assessment tool and a summary copy of the National Cholesterol Education Program–Adult Treatment Panel III (ATP III) guidelines and amendment. The risk assessment tool frequently used is the Framingham Global Coronary Heart Risk Assessment form. This form uses age, sex, smoking history, and blood pressure along with total cholesterol to estimate cardiovascular risk over 10 years. Patients can be placed into low-risk (<10%), intermediate-risk (10%–20%) and high-risk (>20%) categories.

The risk assessment, fasting lipid profile, and ATP III guidelines provide the basic information needed to decide the LDL-C target goals, which is the first focus of treatment. Familiarity with these tools is necessary and will streamline decision making. The treatment of those categorized as low-risk is usually straightforward and consists of lifestyle recommendations, reassurance, and appropriate follow-up.

The high-risk group are those who have known CAD or CAD risk equivalents, or a greater than 20% 10-year risk. This group requires treatment, most often initiated with a statin. Management decisions will focus on how aggressive treatment should be to achieve the greatest patient benefit. The amendment to the ATP III guidelines [13] allows an LDL-C treatment goal of 70 mg/dL for patients at the highest risk based on physician judgment.

Specific recommendations for patients in the intermediate-risk group present a greater challenge. Patients in this group can be divided into symptomatic and asymptomatic [14–32].

Patients who have symptoms require further testing, such as stress testing with or without imaging, electron-beam computerized tomography, 64-slice CT, or coronary angiography with or without IVUS. The goal is to determine whether symptoms are secondary to CAD. The appropriate choice, balancing cost and patient risk, is often complex and frequently requires the opinion of a cardiologist or physician knowledgeable in this area.

Recommendations for patients who have no symptoms in the intermediate-risk group may be even more challenging. For instance, a 45-year-old man or 55-year-old woman who has a strong family history of CAD and some mild hypertension controlled with a small dose of a single antihypertensive but is totally asymptomatic would be in the intermediate-risk group (10%–20% risk). Deciding whether to investigate further or simply follow up is not always easy. A "one decision fits all" approach clearly does not apply to this group, and keen clinical judgment, including the patient's input, is necessary [14].

Treatment: diet and exercise

Diet and exercise are the foundation of any treatment and should be emphasized in all patients who have dyslipidemia. Physicians and staff generally do not have the time, inclination, or expertise to provide detailed dietary advice. Therefore, it may be prudent to enlist the services of a dietician. Clinical staff should emphasize the importance of a proper diet. A cardiac rehabilitation program can help guide eligible patients in developing a proper exercise program. Those who do not qualify for formal cardiac rehabilitation may enroll in community programs through other institutions, such as the hospital or YMCA.

However, valuable time may be lost in starting medication while patients promise to try harder and do better next time with diet and exercise. This phenomenon is well known as the "treatment gap." Unfortunately, as valuable as diet and exercise can be, they often will not bring the patient's LDL-C to goal. Therefore, it may be wiser to start medicine along with diet and exercise. Medicine can always be decreased or stopped if success is accomplished through other means.

Treatment with statins

A statin is the first drug to consider in almost all patients who have significant risk or known atherosclerotic cardiovascular disease. Statins are generally well tolerated, have a high degree of safety, and are the most effective drugs in lowering LDL-C and decreasing events. All statins are 3-hydroxy-3-methlglutaryl coenzyme A reductase inhibitors and act by upgrading the LDL receptors in the liver to increase the metabolism of LDL-C. Some differences exist in solubility, duration of action, and method of metabolism, but the biggest clinical difference between statins is in the relative potency in LDL-C lowering.

Based on current information, the choice of statin should allow the goal to be achieved using a moderate dose. The approximate equivalent doses of statin are fluvastatin, 80 mg = lovastatin, 40 mg = pravastatin, 40 mg = simvastatin, 20 mg = atorvastatin, 10 mg = rosuvastatin, 5 mg. To avoid possible toxic effects from choosing the highest dose of a given statin, some clinicians choose a moderate dose of a more potent statin to achieve the desired amount of LDL-C lowering.

The percent lowering of LDL-C that can be expected varies considerably: 20% to 35% from the weaker statins to 30% to 65% from the more potent statins. The statins all have a mild to moderate effect on lowering triglycerides and improving HDL-C. Statins are generally metabolized by the CYP450-3A4 enzyme system (except fluvastatin, pravastatin, and rosuvastatin). Drugs that interfere or inhibit this system may allow elevated or toxic levels of statins to occur. For example, the dose of simvastatin should be limited to 20 mg or less when used with amiodarone.

When upward titrating a statin, the LDL-C usually lowers approximately 6% each time the dose is doubled [23]. This effect generally occurs for each statin and is a useful guide. If, for example, the current dose of statin is simvastatin, 40 mg, and the goal is to lower the LDL-C another 20%, increasing simvastatin to 80 mg is probably ineffective and another more potent statin should be considered, such as atorvastatin or rosuvastatin as monotherapy. If possible, monotherapy is preferred for safety, cost, and lack of large trials confirming efficacy of combination therapy. However, some high-risk patients will not be able to experience adequate LDL-C lowering without combination therapy.

Probably the most commonly used combination for LDL-C lowering is ezetimibe with any statin. The combination of simvastatin (in all strengths) plus ezetimibe is marketed as Vytorin. Ezetimibe has a good safety record and seems to be well tolerated. Although it is weak by itself, it can have a 17% LDL-C lowering effect when added to a statin [23,26].

Other drugs that have LDL-C lowering effects are resins and niacin. Bile acid sequestrants (cholestyramine, colesevelam, colestipol) are resins and can be used alone or in combination with a statin. Although considered safe, they require several daily doses and cause side effects of bloating and constipation.

Treatment with niacin

Niacin actually does all things that are good for the lipid profile. As monotherapy it lowers triglycerides moderately (25%–30%), decreases LDL-C mildly (14%), and increases HDL-C (25%). Unfortunately, the older, less-expensive, short-acting niacin preparations at effective doses frequently caused side effects of flushing, headache, nausea, rash, and itching. Niacin could also be hepatotoxic, cause hyperuricemia, and worsen diabetic control. Therefore, immediate-release niacin is unpopular among physicians.

Extended-release niacin is much more tolerable, and the newer formulation is even more so. Taken at night, with a small low-fat snack and 81 to 325 mg of aspirin, makes it even more tolerable. The dosage is 500 mg to 2000 mg slowly titrated over 3 to 4 months. Niacin is superior to other currently available drugs in increasing HDL-C, and the combination of a statin and niacin is effective and acceptably safe. In combination with a moderate dose of a statin, niacin reduces LDL-C by 40% and increases HDL-C by 30%.

Treatment with fibrates

Fibrates are not prescribed primarily to lower LDL-C and should not be prescribed unless triglycerides are elevated or HDL-C is low. However, fibrates are frequently used in combination with a statin after the LDL-C is at goal to improve the HDL-C or lower triglycerides. They may also be used in combination with extended-release niacin in patients whose triglycerides and HDL-C cannot be brought to acceptable levels with monotherapy.

Treatment with resins

Resins bind bile acids in the intestine, stimulating the synthesis of cholesterol in the liver, and increasing LDL receptors in the liver, promoting removal of LDL-C from the plasma. Generally safe, they lower cholesterol only moderately as monotherapy (10%–25%), but may be used with other cholesterol-lowering agents. They should not be prescribed in patients who have high triglycerides. Resins have some disadvantages: multiple daily doses are often required, some products require mixing powder with liquids, and all can cause annoying gastrointestinal side effects [33].

Safety of lipid-lowering drugs

Statin safety

As a class, the statins have been remarkably safe; however, like any medicine, they are not 100% safe and the risk–benefit ratio must always be in favor of the patient. The general public has concerns about the muscles and liver and about cancer and Alzheimer's disease. Muscle complaints are most common. Subgroups of patients that are more likely to experience symptoms include patients who have diabetics, small underweight women, the elderly, and those on polypharmacy.

Muscle symptoms

Currently, the definition of statin-related muscle complaints is not standardized. Therefore, muscle problems are difficult to define when data collection varies from study to study. The Expert Muscle Panel of the National Lipid Association (NLA) has recommended a standardized format for data collection and clinical use. An in-depth review of this topic and other safety issues can be found in the *American Journal of Cardiology* [34]. Statins have been associated with three main adverse symptoms affecting muscle: myalgia, myopathy, and rhabdomyolysis.

- Myalgia: Muscle aches, pain or weakness with or without creatine kinase (CK) elevation.

- Myopathy: Unexplained elevation of CK greater than 10 times the upper normal limit associated with muscle symptoms.
- Rhabdomyolysis: Marked elevation of CK greater than 10 times the upper normal limit with elevation of serum creatinine and renal insufficiency, requiring hydration, hospitalization, and usually nephrology consultation. Up to 50% may not have muscle symptoms.

With myalgias, the muscle aches but no abnormal physical findings are present and the creatine kinase (CK) is less than 10,000. Mild elevations in CK are common in active people, and elevation in the 100s or even low 1000s can occur after vigorous exercise, such as running. These low level elevations in CK can usually be ignored and therapy continued.

A baseline CK before treatment with a statin is usually not needed or routinely recommended. However, baseline CKs may be considered in high-risk groups, such as the elderly and those on polypharmacy, combination lipid therapy, and drugs known to increase the levels of statins, such as erythromycin, itraconazole/ketoconazole, or cyclosporine. If simvastatin or lovastatin are prescribed with either amiodarone or verapamil, it should be at the lowest doses.

Myalgias are often a variable and tolerable nuisance, and are more frequently seen in the older population. However, for some individuals, myalgias become genuinely intolerable despite having normal or acceptably normal CKs. In these patients, the statin should be reduced or frequently switched to another. Sometimes reducing the statin to every other or every third day may be effective. High-risk patients who can clearly benefit from a statin yet remain intolerant may need to omit the drug for several weeks and then return to therapy. Difficult to manage patients may need to be referred to a lipid clinic. With patience and understanding from the health care provider and a spirit of cooperation, most patients requiring a statin can tolerate one.

Myopathy is diffuse muscle symptoms of large muscle groups and CKs that are greater than 10 times the upper normal limit. The offending drug should be stopped until the symptoms resolve and, depending on the need for the lipid–lowering, another statin tried with careful monitoring.

Rhabdomyolysis is a serious and potentially fatal disease. It may occur at any time (early or late) when taking a statin. Muscle pain often occurs, but not always. CKs are elevated to greater than 10,000 and dark urine (myoglobinuria), elevation in the serum creatinine, and possible renal failure may be present. Treatment requires discontinuation of the statin and hospitalization with intravenous hydration. The morality rate is approximately 10%. This serious and potentially fatal reaction to statin therapy is fortunately very rare. Best estimates are one occurrence in 15 million prescriptions. Also, on the positive side, statins in combination with extended-release niacin, a bile acid resin, ezetimibe, omega 3 fatty acid, a plant sterol, or stanols seem to cause no increase in myopathy or rhabdomyolysis compared with a statin alone.

Liver disease

Although statins are well known to be associated with an increase in liver enzymes (transaminases), the bigger question is whether these elevations are meaningful. Increase in aminotransaminase (AST) and alanine transferase (ALT) greater than three times the upper limit normal occurs in less than 1% of patients taking a statin at the low- or mid-dose (ie, <80 mg). At the 80 mg dose, elevation of AST and ALT greater than three times the upper limit normal occurs in 1% to 3% of patients. If enzymes are repeated, these elevations are found to be transient and resolve without treatment 70% of the time despite continued therapy [2]. The NLA Statin Safety Task Force has concluded that liver enzymes are often transiently elevated with statin therapy and that liver failure rarely, if ever, occurs in patients taking statins, and no more often than in the general population [35].

Despite evidence that monitoring liver enzymes offers little safety for patients, the FDA requires transaminase studies be obtained before and during statin therapy. These studies must be performed according to the package insert instructions until the FDA requirements change.

The Expert Liver Panel [2,36] also believes that statins are safe in nonalcoholic steatohepatitis, nonalcoholic fatty liver, chronic liver disease, and compensated cirrhosis. Statins are contraindicated in decompensated cirrhosis or acute liver failure.

Cancer

From the early development of statins and their effect on lowering cholesterol, a theoretic concern existed about a risk for cancer. However, clinical trials have not provided data implicating statins in causing cancer.

Alzheimer's disease and neuropathy

The NLA Neurology Expert Panel [37,38] found no causal relationship between impaired memory and cognitive function and statin therapy.

To summarize, and put into perspective the safety of statins, the NLA performed an analysis showing that for every million people who have a high cholesterol level, a statin reduces heart attacks, strokes, and revascularizations in approximately 10,000, whereas only one or two will experience a serious, life-threatening adverse effect.

Safety of nonstatins

Fibrate safety

Renal insufficiency

The class of fibrates may infrequently cause an increase in creatinine level, although this apparently does not represent renal damage. Creatinine clearance does not decrease, despite the increase in creatinine. Fibrates should be used at lower doses in individuals who have renal dysfunction and should not be used in patients undergoing renal dialysis because of the narrow margin between effective and toxic doses.

Myopathy and rhabdomyolysis

Fibrates as monotherapy may cause myopathy and rhabdomyolysis, but rarely. In combination with a statin, the incidence is low, but is significantly increased with gemfibrozil. When combining with a statin, the preferred fibrate is fenofibrate. Because statins and fibrates can both cause myopathy individually, avoiding the maximum dose of statin is recommended when these are used in combination.

Niacin safety

Flushing, rash, and erythema

Flushing occurs in 66% of individuals taking immediate-release niacin [29]. This side effect leads to frequent discontinuation of effective doses; extended-release niacin is much more tolerable. Nevertheless, a feeling of flushing, warmth, and occasionally erythema is not uncommon. "No-flush" and "flush-free" niacin are currently marketed; however, no evidence shows that this formulation increases circulating niacin or alters

plasma lipids. Therefore, niacin does not seem to be bioavailable in this form. Alcohol and hot and spicy foods can cause increased flushing and may require timed dosing.

Myopathy and rhabdomyolysis

Niacin monotherapy does not cause myopathy, rhabdomyolysis, or CK elevation. Combination therapy with niacin and a statin does not cause muscle adverse experience compared with statins alone.

Diabetic control

Niacin can infrequently worsen diabetic control. Current formulations seem to cause less hyperglycemia than older preparations, but should be monitored.

Hyperuricemia

A mild increase in uric acid occurs, but still within normal range and does not seem to be the problem of older preparations.

Ezetimibe safety

Ezetimibe is a gastrointestinal-active drug that seems safe and has the adverse event rate of placebo in clinical trials. It is approved for use with statins and fibrates.

The importance of high-density lipoprotein cholesterol

Almost all health care providers and most health-conscious individuals are aware of "good" cholesterol (HDL-C) and "bad" cholesterol (LDL-C). Although this simple terminology is still meaningful for LDL-C, the situation is much more complex for HDL-C. Normally, HDL-C is considered protective, and in fact a value greater than 60 mg/dL allows the subtraction of one point on the Framingham risk assessment. However, sometimes HDL-C can change from protective to unprotective or can become inflammatory.

The common belief that increased HDL-C protects against cardiovascular risk is untrue. A recent clinical trial with a cholesterol ester transfer protein inhibitor was halted early because of increased cardiovascular deaths despite a marked increase in the HDL-C. The issues are complex, but simply increasing HDL-C does not seem to protect against risk; this may be more from the functionality of the HDL-C than the actual amount. Currently, treating patients at risk for increased LDL-C with a statin is considered reasonable, even though the HDL-C may be high, because no practical clinical test exists to evaluate the functionality of the HDL-C.

For individuals who require a statin and still have a low HDL-C, treating with combination therapy through adding niacin or a fibrate seems appropriate. The post hoc analysis of the Treat to New Targets trial showed that low HDL-C values still predicted risk in individuals who had LDL-C less than 70 mg/dL treated with atorvastatin. This finding seems to support treating at-risk patients with statin and niacin if the HDL-C is low [39–43].

The value of non–high-density lipoprotein cholesterol

Although LDL-C can be measured directly, the value obtained on the standard blood lipid is a value calculated from the measured total cholesterol, HDL-C, and triglycerides using the Friedewald equation. When triglyceride values are greater than 200 mg/dL, the formula becomes inaccurate for calculating LDL-C, thereby losing the accuracy of the main target for lipid lowering.

Non–HDL-C is simply subtracting the HDL-C value from the total cholesterol. This value reflects the amount of arthrogenic particles and is a secondary target when the LDL-C is inaccurate or the triglycerides are greater than 200 mg/dL.

The desired value for non–HDL-C is 30 mg/dL higher than the target LDL-C (ie, if a LDL-C of 70 mg/dL is the goal for a high-risk patient, the non–HDL-C goal is 100 mg/dL). This calculation is valuable and simple, and is particularly helpful in managing those who have hypertriglyceridemia.

Women and heart disease

CAD is the leading cause of mortality and morbidity in the United States. Since 1984, more women have died of ischemic heart disease than men, and it is the cause of death in more than 250,000 women each year [40]. Women's cardiovascular mortality increases with age, whereas men's mortality decreases.

Women at angioplasty have less obstructive CAD, but for the given amount their prognosis seems worse. These observations suggest that more functional abnormalities may be present compared with men. Perhaps the abnormality is at the microvascular level. Historically, women have been treated similarly to men, with guidelines

developed from clinical trials that included few women.

Women's symptoms have been noted to be more dyspnea and fatigue than chest tightness. The frequency of false-positive treadmill stress tests in women has never been convincingly explained. Until further information is available, no reason exists to alter the current guidelines. Currently, symptomatic women must be viewed with concern and not ignored. Lifestyle changes and prudent use of statins, ace inhibitors, and aspirin should be encouraged.

Progress in lipid therapy over the past decade?

The first survey, the Lipid Treatment Assessment Program, was completed in 1996/1997 [41]. This study showed that 38% patients overall and 18% who had CAD had achieved the ATP III goals. In 2001, the ATP III guidelines were adopted, with an additional amendment that included the option to treat high-risk patients to a LDL-C of 70 mg/dL [14]. Five new statins were developed in the 1900s and one in 2003. The newer statins are more effective in lowering LDL-C without significant increase in side effects, making the goal easier to achieve with monotherapy.

Neptune II was a 2003 national survey of the top 26% prescribers of statins (internists, family physicians, and specialists) [42]. This survey showed that 68% of patients achieved goal, and 62% who had CAD achieved an LDL-C level less than 100 mg/dL. However, only 55% who had diabetes, 40% who had CAD risk equivalents, and 40% who had a greater than 20% 10-year risk for CAD were at goal. Only 27% were achieving the goal of LDL-C and non–HDL-C with triglycerides of greater than 200 mg/dL. The study was probably biased for overachieving, because the group consisted of aggressive prescribers of statins.

The National Health and Nutrition Examination Survey in 1999/2000 indicated that only 35% of patients who had elevated cholesterol were aware of it and 12% were treated; 36.5 million qualify for drug treatment with ATP III guidelines, only 11 million receive it, and only a portion are to effective goals [42].

Summary

The proof that drug therapy can reduce mortality and cardiac events is now beyond question.

Drug therapy, particularly the statins, is effective and acceptably safe in qualified patients. Simple information from a fasting lipid profile, a coronary risk assessment tool, and ATP guidelines provide an effective working model for treatment. Despite abundant information available to the public and medical professionals, there are many people who are at risk who do not know their cholesterol levels, have not been treated, or are ineffectively treated. Empowering an educated nursing staff, who is more frequently the first point of contact, to appropriately initiate assessment and treatment guidelines, under the guidance of their supervising physician should impact this treatment gap.

References

[1] Topol EJ. Intensive statin therapy—a sea change in cardiovascular prevention. N Engl J Med 2004;350: 1562–4.

[2] Gotto MG. Statins, cardiovascular disease, and drug safety. Am J Cardiol 2006;97(Suppl):3C–5C.

[3] Heart Protection Study Collaborative Group. MRC/BHF Heart Protection Study of cholesterol lowering with simvastatin in 20, 536 high-risk individuals: a randomised placebo-controlled trial. Lancet 2002;360(9236):7–22.

[4] Scandinavian Simvastatin Survival Study Group. Randomised trail of cholesterol lowing in 4444 patients with coronary heart disease: the Scandinavian Simvastatin Survival Study (4S). Lancet 1994;344: 1383–9.

[5] Gotto MG. Review of primary and secondary prevention trials with lovastatin, pravastatin and simvastatin. Am J Cardiol 2005;96(Suppl):34F–8F.

[6] Gurm HS, Hoogwerf B. The heart protection study: high-risk patients benefit from statins, regardless of LDL-C level. Cleve Clin J Med 2003;70(11):991–7.

[7] Bose D, von Birgelen C, Erbel R. Intravascular ultrasound for the evaluation of therapies targeting coronary atherosclerosis. J Am Coll Cardiol 2007; 49:925–32.

[8] Nissen SE. For the reversal investigators effect of intensive compared with moderate lipid-lowering therapy on progression of coronary atherosclerosis. JAMA 2004;291:1071–80.

[9] Nissen SE. Effect of lipid lowering on progression of atherosclerosis: evidence for an early benefit from the reversal of atherosclerosis with aggressive lipid lowering (REVERSAL). Am J Cardiol 2005; 96(Suppl):61F–8F.

[10] Klein LW. Atherosclerosis regression, vascular remodeling, and plaque stabilization. J Am Coll Cardiol 2007;49:271–3.

[11] Nissen SE, ASTEROID Investigators. Effect of very high-intensity statin therapy on regression of coronary atherosclerosis the asteroid trial. JAMA 2006;295:1556–65.

[12] Sipahi I, Nicholls SJ, Tuzcu EM, et al. Coronary atherosclerosis can regress with very intensive statin therapy. Cleve Clin J Med 2006;73:937–44.

[13] Grundy SM, Cleeman H, Merz CN, et al. Implications of recent clinical trials for the National Cholesterol Education Program Adult Treatment Panel III Guidelines. Circulation 2004;110:227–39.

[14] Executive summary of the third report of the national cholesterol education program (NCEP) expert panel on detection, evaluation, and treatment of high blood cholesterol in adults (Adult Treatment Panel III). JAMA 2001;285:2496–7.

[15] Merz NB. Assessment of patients at intermediate cardiac risk. Am J Cardiol 2005;96(Suppl):2J–10J.

[16] Product information brochure Lescol prescribing information. Novartis Pharmaceuticals, May 2003.

[17] Mevacor prescribing information, Merck and Co., Inc., April 2005.

[18] Pravachol prescribing information, Bristol-Meyers Squibb Co., December 2004.

[19] Zocor prescribing information, Merck and Co., Inc., November 2004.

[20] Lipitor prescribing information, Pfizer Ireland Pharmaceuticals, July 2004.

[21] Crestor prescribing information, AstraZenica Pharmaceuticals, March 2005.

[22] [Product information brochure]. Merck and Co., Inc.

[23] Hutter AM, Jones PH, Plutzky J. Combination therapies for cholesterol management ACC conversations with experts. 2004 Text compendium.

[24] Niaspan [product information brochure]. Miami (FL): Kos Pharmaceuticals; 2007.

[25] Advicor [product information brochure]. Miami (FL): Kos Pharmaceuticals; 2006.

[26] Zetia [product information brochure]. Whitehouse Station (NJ): Merck & Co.; 2005.

[27] Davidson MJ. APPOLLO Advances in prevention through optimal lipid lowering newsletter volume 4, 2007.

[28] Davidson MJ, Armani A, McKenney JM, et al. Safety considerations with fibrate therapy. Am J Cardiol 2007;99(Suppl):3C–16C.

[29] Guyton JR, Bays HE. Safety considerations with niacin therapy. Am J Cardiol 2007;99(Suppl): 22C–31C.

[30] Toth PP. Expert commentary: gastrointestinally active lipid-lowering drug safety. Am J Cardiol 2007; 99(Suppl):56C–8C.

[31] Nissen SE, Tardif JC, Nicholls SJ, et al. Effect of torcetrapib on the progression of coronary atherosclerosis. N Engl J Med 2007;356:1304–16.

[32] Freidwalk VE, Brewer BH, Grundy SM, et al. The editor's roundtable: high-density lipoprotein cholesterol. Am J Cardiol 2007;99:1698–705.

[33] Jacobson TA, Armani A, McKenney JM, et al. Safety considerations with gastrointestinally active

lipid-lowering drugs. Am J Cardiol 2007;99(6A): 47C–55C.

[34] Thompson PD, Clarkson PM, Rosenson RS. An assessment of statin safety by muscle experts. Am J Cardiol 2006;97(8A):69C–76C.

[35] Jacobson TA. Statin safety: lessons from new drug applications for marketed statins. Am J Cardiol 2006;97(8A):44C–51C.

[36] Cohen DE, Anania FA, Chalasani N. An assessment of statin safety by hepatologists. Am J Cardiol 2006; 97(8A):77C–81C.

[37] Brass LM, Alperts MJ, Sparks L. An assessment of statin safety by neurologists. Am J Cardiol 2006; 97(8A):86C–8C.

[38] McKenney JM, Davidson MH, Jacobson TA, et al. Final conclusions and recommendations of the National Lipid Association Statin Safety Assessment Task Force. Am J Cardiol 2006;97(8A): 89C–94C.

[39] Barter P, Gotto AM, LaRosa JC, et al. HDL cholesterol, very low levels of LDL cholesterol and cardiovascular events. N Engl J Med 2007; 357:1301–10.

[40] Jacobs AK. Women, ischemic heart disease, revascularization, and the gender gap what are we missing? J Am Coll Cardiol 2006;47(Suppl):63S–5S.

[41] Pearson TA, Laurora I, Chu H, et al. The Lipid Treatment Assessment Project (L-Tap): a multi-center survey to evaluate the percentages of dyslipidemia patients receiving lipid-lowering lipoprotein cholesterol goals. Arch Intern Med 2000;160: 459–67.

[42] Davidson MH, Maki KC, Pearson TA, et al. Results of the National Cholesterol Education (NCEP) Program Evaluation Project Utilizing Novel E Technology (NEPTUNE) II survey and implications for treatment under the recent NCEP writing group recommendations. Am J Cardiol 2005;96:556–663.

[43] Erhardt LR. Barriers to effective implementation of guidelines recommendations. Am J Med 2005; 118(Suppl 12A):36S–41S.

CRITICAL CARE
NURSING CLINICS
OF NORTH AMERICA

Common Obstacles in Lipid Management

Missie Elpers, MS

The Heart Group, 415 West Columbia Street, Evansville, Indiana 47710, USA

The importance of lipid management with the use of statins and other cholesterol medications are quite clear. For most individuals, the ability to manage lipid levels with adjustments in lifestyle and the use of cholesterol-altering medications is not complicated. A smaller group of individuals is more challenging to treat because of their reluctance to take medications, their sensitivity to medications, or the complexity of starting certain medications. Table 1 outlines the common medications used in lipid management.

Managing lipids in these challenging individuals is more time consuming and frustrating for physicians, practitioners, and support staff. Often, this challenge leads to patients not being treated appropriately to achieve their target lipid levels or not being treated at all.

Spending more time initially in educating patients about their treatment plan and addressing their concerns leads to better compliance and fewer difficulties later. Simply handing a patient a few medication samples and a prescription may not be the most effective treatment approach. The last thing a skeptical patient needs is an unwanted surprise from the new medication or treatment plan.

Why are some patients noncompliant with their cholesterol medications? The number of reasons seems endless to many health care providers. The biggest patient-related obstacles in treating lipid disorders seem to be a patient's fear of statins, a patient's sensitivity to or intolerance to statins, and the patient's inability to withstand the side effects of starting niacin.

Some patients believe the benefits of taking a statin to control their cholesterol are not worth the risks they may incur by not taking the medication. Patients' reluctance to take these medications results in part from their lack of understanding of what the drug can do for them and of the real risks from the complications of hyperlipidemia. The media and patient advocacy groups have exaggerated and provided misinformation about the side effects of statins [1].

It is important for patients to be aware of side effects of all of their medications, but it is not in patients' best interest to make them afraid to take medications. Many physicians and nonphysicians know that statins can cause muscle aches and weakness. Unfortunately, patients interpret these symptoms as indicating permanent debilitating muscle damage. Myalgias defined as muscle pain, weakness, or stiffness without creatine phosphokinase (CPK) elevation is a common but not a serious side effect of statins. These symptoms generally resolve when the use of the statin is discontinued. On the other hand, myositis and rhabdomyositis present with the same type of symptoms but with CPK levels elevated more than 10 times the upper limit of normal. These serious conditions should be ruled out when symptoms of muscle aches or weakness present. Fortunately, these conditions are rare [2]. Patients should be instructed to report any muscle aches, weakness, stiffness, or brown urine immediately, and a CPK level should be drawn so further treatment can be implemented if indicated. If myositis or rhabdomyositis is suspected or diagnosed, statin treatment should be stopped immediately [3].

Patients also are afraid statins will cause liver damage and tend to be more worried about liver health than about cholesterol levels or heart health. In reality, statins are safe medications and are not likely to cause progressive liver disease [4]. Hepatotoxicity is detected by an increase in transaminase

E-mail address: missie22@heartgroup.com

Table 1
Medications used in lipid management

Medication and dose	Effect	Practice pearls
HMG CoA reductase inhibitors (statins): take at night Atorvastatin (Lipitor), 10–80 mg/d Fluvastatin (Lescol), 20–80 mg/d Lovastatin (Mevacor), 20–80 mg/d Lovastatin (Altoprev extended release), 60 mg/d Pravastatin (Pravachol), 10–80 mg/d Simvastatin (Zocor), 5 mg d; 40/d mg for patients who have CAD or DM Rosuvastatin (Crestor), 10–40 mg/d	↓ LDL 18%–55% ↑ HDL 5%–15% ↓ Triglycerides 7%–30%	Check hepatic enzymes (LFTs) before initiation, at 3 months after starting or changing dose, and then periodically every 6–12 months; stop drug if levels are three times normal. Check CK at initiation to establish baseline. Ongoing evaluation in the absence of symptoms is not warranted. Adverse effects: rhabdomyolysis and myositis are rare but are noted most often with higher statin dosages.
Bile acid sequestrants/resins Cholestyramine, (Questran, Cholybar), 4 g tid or qid Colestipol, (Colestid) 6 g/d Colesevelam (Welchol), three tablets bid or six tablets qd with food	↓ LDL 15%–30% ↑ HDL 3%–5%	No hepatic monitoring required. Minimal effect on triglycerides. Adverse effects: Gastrointestinal distress, constipation, decreased absorption of other drugs if taken within 2 hours of many medications
Nicotinic acid Niacin, 1–3 g tid with or after meals Niaspan (extended release), 500 mg hs, adjust dose by 500 mg/d at 4-week intervals	↑ HDL 15%–35% ↓ Triglycerides 20%–50% ↓ LDL 5%–25%	Particularly effective against highly atherogenic lipoprotein. Adverse effects: Flushing (may take aspirin or Motrin 30 minutes before taking niacin to reduce flushing), hyperglycemia, hyperuricemia, upper gastrointestinal tract distress, hepatotoxicity. Contraindications: Active liver disease, severe gout, peptic ulcer disease
Fibric acid derivatives (fibrates) Gemfibrozil (Lopid), 600 mg bid ac Fenofibrate (Tricor), 67–200 mg/d Clofibrate (Atromid-S), 2 g/d	↑ HDL 10%–20% ↓ Triglycerides 20%–50% ↓ LDL 5%–20%	Adverse effects: Dyspepsia, gallstones, myopathy including rhabdomyolysis if taken with a statin. Contraindicated in severe renal or hepatic disease.
Ezetimibe (Zetia), 10 mg/d	↓ LDL 15%–20% ↑ HDL 3%–5%	Minimal effect on triglycerides. Most often prescribed with another lipid-lowering agent such as a statin to enhance LDL reduction. Adverse effects: Few because of limited systemic absorption.
Fish oil (omega-3 fatty acid) Omacor, 4 g/d	↓ Triglycerides 20%–30% ↑ HDL 1%–5%	Refrigerate to decrease "fishy" taste. Adverse effects: Gastrointestinal upset and increased risk of bleeding.

Abbreviations: ac, before meal; CAD, coronary artery disease; CK, creatinine kinase; DM, diabetes mellitus; HDL, high-density lipoprotein; hs, at bedtime; LDL, low-density lipoprotein.

Data from Adult Treatment Panel III (ATP III) guidelines, National Cholesterol Education Program. Available at: http://www.nhlbi.nih.gov/guidelines/cholesterol/atglance.pdf. Accessed December 2007.

levels, with a reported frequency of only1%, usually when patients are taking other hepatotoxic medications or consume alcohol regularly in addition to their statin medication. Statin discontinuation is not recommended unless the transaminase levels exceed three times the normal limits. Once the elevated transaminase levels return to baseline, statin therapy can be reinitiated at a lower dose, or a different statin may be prescribed [2,5].

Lipid-clinic physicians and lipid-specialist educators need to spend time building patients' confidence and reducing their fears about the use of statins. It must be explained to the patients that statin medications are the drugs of choice to lower low-density lipoprotein (LDL) cholesterol levels because of their potency and their ability to stabilize plaques and to reduce cardiovascular and stroke events [6]. Patients need to be educated about the differences between myalgias and myositis and the steps that will be taken to distinguish and treat the two conditions. For patients who fear liver damage, it also is helpful to explain briefly how the medications work in the liver to lower cholesterol levels. Patients should be assured that their liver function test (LFT) will be checked before statin initiation to screen for any indications that would contraindicate the use of the medication and that their LFT will be checked every 2 to 6 months as long as they remain on the medication. Patients should be instructed to report any medication changes, so drug interactions that may cause an increase in liver enzymes can be reviewed. Sometimes it may be necessary to change lipid medications or alter the dose to avoid a potential problem. The bile acid sequestrants/resins are nonsystemic cholesterol-altering agents that do not affect hepatic function at all. Although these medications are not as potent as statins, they sometimes are the only medications that the patient is willing to take.

Based on what they know and what they have been told, patients certainly have legitimate concerns about taking cholesterol medication. It is important for the health care provider to explain the benefits of the treatment plan and the patient's true risk for developing coronary artery disease. It is hoped that the patient will agree that the benefits outweigh any risk and will allow the health care provider to initiate the appropriate treatment plan. Some patients may be willing to take a lower dose of a statin. This is certainly a good option, especially with the availability of gastrointestinal agents (eg, ezetimibe and resins) that can be used in conjunction with a statin to reduce the LDL cholesterol level to an acceptable range [1].

If all efforts at education fail, and the patient still refuses statin therapy, the practitioner should consider using a gastrointestinal-active agent. Resins are the only nonsystemic lipid agents that will not cause myalgias or affect hepatic function. This advantage seems to be appealing to some statin-phobic patients who may be willing to try this option. Although these medications are not as potent as statins, they sometimes are the only lipid-lowering medication that a practitioner can convince a patient to take.

The issue of statin sensitivity is the principle reason primary care physicians refer patients to a lipid clinic. In general, patients who have reported side effects from various statins tend to have sensitivities to more than one drug. When treating patients, one should be cognizant that elderly patients, those who have multiple system failure or renal or hepatic insufficiency, patients taking other medications with potential drug interactions, patients who have hypothyroidism, those who drink excessive amounts of alcohol, and those who have electrolyte imbalances or dehydration are at increased risk of developing myalgias or myopathy [3,7]. The health care provider must make additional efforts to find a treatment plan that works for a statin-sensitive patient. For patients who clearly would benefit from a statin, it is important not to give up too quickly on all statin options and label these patients as statin intolerant. Patients who experience side effects from one or more statins may not be intolerant to all statins.

A health care provider should evaluate thoroughly each patient's complaints about medication. Too often the mention of muscle aches, stiffness, or cramps leads to a hasty decision to stop the use of the statin and to list the patient as intolerant to the medication [8]. At times the statin is the cause of the patient's symptoms, but there are times when the patient's symptoms have a different cause, such as the addition of physical activity, a recent injury or accident, a different medication, or new medical condition. If the patient's symptoms do not resolve with discontinuation of the statin, other causes should be investigated, and reinitiating the statin should be considered. If the patient's symptoms resolve after medication discontinuation, it certainly is reasonable to consider restarting use of the medication at a lower dose or changing to a different medication [9].

Finding a treatment plan for patients who are sensitive to statins but who would benefit from

Table 2
Characteristics of the various statins[a]

Characteristic	Lovastatin (Mevacor)	Pravastatin (Pravachol)	Simvastatin (Zocor)	Fluvastatin (Lescol)	Atorvastatin (Lipitor)	Rosuvastatin (Crestor)
Dosage and average per cent decrease in LDL cholesterol	20 mg: 29 40 mg: 31 80 mg: 40–48	10 mg: 19 20 mg: 24 40 mg: 34 80 mg: 40	10 mg: 28 20 mg: 35 40 mg: 40 80 mg: 48	20 mg: 17 40 mg: 23 80 mg: 33	10 mg: 38 20 mg: 46 40 mg: 51 80 mg: 54	5 mg: 43 10 mg: 50 20 mg: 53 40 mg: 62
Renal function	Use lower doses when there is severe renal impairment (creatinine clearance < 30 mL/min). Use caution with doses > 20mg/d.	Use lower doses when there is significant renal impairment; reduce initial dose to 10 mg/d).	Use lower doses when there is severe renal impairment; reduce initial dose to 5 mg/d. Canadian labeling advises caution with doses > 10 mg/d.	No dose adjustment necessary for reduced renal function (not studied at doses > 40 mg in severe renal impairment). Use not advised in severe impairment per Canadian labeling.	No dose adjustment necessary for reduced renal function. Canadian labeling recommends the lowest dose (10 mg/d) for moderate/severe renal insufficiency.	Use lower doses for severe renal impairment (creatinine clearance < 30 mL/min not to exceed 10 mg/d.
Liver function monitoring	LFTs at baseline, before doses > 40 mg/d, and periodically or when clinically indicated	LFTs at baseline, before elevation of dose, and when otherwise clinically indicated. Canadian labeling also recommends LFTs 12 weeks after starting therapy and after dose increase.	LFTs at baseline and thereafter when clinically indicated. Patients titrated to 80 mg should receive an additional test before titration, 3 months after titration, and every 6 months for the first year.	LFTs at baseline and at 12 weeks (8 weeks per Canadian labeling) after initiation or elevation of dose.	LFTs at baseline and at 12 weeks following therapy initiation or dose elevation. Check every 6 months thereafter. Canadian labels advise baseline and periodic LFTs.	LFTs at baseline and 12 weeks after initiation or elevation of dose, then every 6 months thereafter.
Drug interactions	Metabolized by CYP3A4 enzyme system. Watch for interactions with drugs that inhibit this enzyme, including amiodarone, erythromycin, clarithromycin,	Not significantly metabolized by cytochrome P450 and may be less likely to be involved in drug interactions. Cyclosporine can increase pravastatin levels.	Metabolized by CYP3A4 enzyme system. Watch for interactions with drugs that inhibit this enzyme including amiodarone, erythromycin, clarithromycin,	Metabolized primarily by CYP2C9 enzyme system and may be less likely to be involved in drug interactions. Fluvastatin can increase levels of phenytoin. Rifampin can lower fluvastatin	Metabolized by CYP3A4 enzyme system, but less so than lovastatin and simvastatin. Drugs that inhibit CYP3A4 include erythromycin, clarithromycin, ketoconazole,	Not significantly metabolized by cytochrome P450 and may be less likely to be involved in drug interactions. Use lower doses with cyclosporine or gemfibrozil. Canadian labeling

ketoconazole, verapamil, diltiazem, nefazodone, fluvoxamine, cyclosporine, grapefruit juice, and others.	ketoconazole, verapamil, diltiazem, nefazodone, fluvoxamine, cyclosporine, grapefruit juice, and others.	ketoconazole, verapamil, diltiazem, nefazodone, fluvoxamine, cyclosporine, grapefruit juice, and others.	levels. Combinations of fluvastatin (80 mg/d) with glyburide can increase levels of both drugs.	verapamil, nefazodone, fluvoxamine, cyclosporine, grapefruit juice, and others.	states the use of rosuvastatin with cyclosporine is contraindicated. Rosuvastatin with warfarin results in increased INR.
Cost/month ($US/$CAN)					
40 mg: $142/$65 (generic available)	40 mg: $143/$43 (generic available)	20 mg: $147/$44 (generic available)	80 mg XL: $110/$41	10 mg: $100/$53	5 mg: $113/$41
Clinical benefit					
Primary prevention of CHD[b]: Reduces first acute coronary event, MI, unstable angina, and revascularization in patients who have average LDL (AFCAPS/TexCAPS). Slows progression of coronary atherosclerosis in CHD[b] (CCAIT, FATS, MARS). Improvement also in carotid arteries (ACAPS).	Primary prevention of CHD[b]: Reduces cardiovascular death, MI, and revascularization in patients who have high LDL and multiple risk factors (WOSCOPS). Secondary prevention of CHD[b]: Reduces recurrent MI, coronary death, revascularization, and stroke/TIA across range of cholesterol levels (CARE, LIPID). Slows progression of coronary atherosclerosis in CHD[b]; improvement also in carotid arteries (REGRESS, PLAC I, PLAC II, KAPS). Failed to show benefit in hypertensive patients (ALL-HATLLT), but	Primary and secondary prevention of CHD[b]: Reduces risk of total mortality, nonfatal MI, stroke, and revascularization in patients at high risk of coronary events,[c] but with normal cholesterol (including LDL < 100 mg/dL, women, diabetes, and peripheral arterial disease) (HPS). Secondary prevention of CHD[b]: Reduces recurrent MI, coronary and total mortality, revascularization, and stroke in patients with high LDL (4S). Slows progression of atherosclerosis in patients who have CHD and normal to	Slows progression of atherosclerosis in patients who have CHD and mild to moderate hypercholesterolemia (LCAS). Secondary prevention of CHD: Reduces risk of revascularization procedures. Dose of 40 mg bid reduced risk of MACE when begun within days after PCI in patients who had average cholesterol levels (LIPS). Did not reduce MACE in renal transplant recipients, but secondary end points of cardiac death and MI were reduced (ALERT). No benefit for early treatment of ACS with 80 mg/d (FLORIDA).	Primary prevention of CHD: Reduces nonfatal MI, fatal CHD, and stroke in patients who have hypertension and total cholesterol < 250 mg/dL (ASCOT). Primary prevention of CHD: Reduces coronary events, revascularization, and stroke in patients who have type 2 diabetes, an additional CHD risk factor, and LDL <160 mg/dL. (CARDS preliminary report). Secondary prevention of CHD: Reduced risk of coronary morbidity and mortality, and stroke in open-label comparison with usual care of patients who had	Regression of atherosclerosis with intensive statin therapy in patients who have angiographic coronary disease. 40mg/d reduced LDL (mean, 60.8 mg/dL), raised HDL (mean, 49.0 mg/dL), reduced percent mean atheroma volume by 0.98% (ASTEROID). Slows progression of atherosclerosis[b] (METEOR)

(continued on next page)

Table 2
Characteristics of the various statins[a]

Characteristic	Lovastatin (Mevacor)	Pravastatin (Pravachol)	Simvastatin (Zocor)	Fluvastatin (Lescol)	Atorvastatin (Lipitor)	Rosuvastatin (Crestor)
		result probably reflects high non-study statin use in usual care group. Preliminary study found lower risk of MACE with early therapy of ACS (L-CAD). Reduced composite of coronary death, nonfatal MI, and stroke in high-risk patients > 70 years old, but no benefit for stroke alone; result attributed to short study duration (PROSPER).	high cholesterol (MAAS, SCAT). Combined with niacin reduces major coronary events in patients who have CHD and HDL < 35 mg/dL (HATS). Reduces vascular events (HPS) and development/progression of intermittent claudication (4S) in peripheral arterial disease.		LDL > 100 mg/dL (GREACE). 80 mg/d begun within 1–4 days after ACS reduced recurrent ischemic events and stroke over 4 months (MIRACL). In ACS, intense lipid lowering (median LDL, 62 mg/dL) reduces risk of death/major cardiovascular events more than moderate lipid lowering (median LDL, 95 mg/dL) (PROVEIT). Regresses/slows progression of atherosclerosis (ASAP, ARBITER, REVERSAL). Unclear benefit in peripheral arterial disease (TREADMILL).	

Abbreviations: ACS, acute coronary syndrome; CHD, coronary heart disease; CYP2C9, cytochrome P-450 2C9; CYP3A4, cytochrome P-450 3A4; HDL, high-density lipoprotein cholesterol; INR, international normalized ratio; LDL, low-density lipoprotein cholesterol; LFT, liver function test; MACE, major adverse cardiac event (cardiac death, non-fatal MI, or revascularization); MI, myocardial infarction; PCI, percutaneous coronary intervention; TIA, transient ischemic attack.

Study acronyms and references:

4S, Scandinavian Simvastatin Survival Study: *Lancet* 1994;344:1383–9. *Am J Cardiol* 1998;81:333–5.

ACAPS, Asymptomatic Carotid Artery Progression Study: *Circulation* 1994;90:1679–87.

AFCAPS/TEXCAPS, Air Force/Texas Coronary Atherosclerosis Prevention Study: *JAMA* 1998;279:1615–22.

ALERT, Assessment of *Lescol* in Renal Transplantation Study: *Lancet* 2003;361:2024–31.

ALLHAT-LLT, Antihypertensive and Lipid-Lowering Treatment to Prevent Heart Attack Trial: *JAMA* 2002;288:2998–3007.

ARBITER, Arterial Biology for the Investigation of the Treatment Effects of Reducing Cholesterol: *Circulation* 2002;106:2055–60.

ASAP, Atorvastatin versus Simvastatin on Atherosclerosis Prevention: *Lancet* 2001;357:577–81.

ASCOT, Anglo-Scandinavian Cardiac Outcomes Trial: *Lancet* 2003;361:1149–58.

ASTEROID, A Study to Evaluate the Effect of Rosuvastatin on Intravascular Ultrasound- Derived Coronary Atheroma Burden: *JAMA* 2006;295:(doi:10.1001/jama.295.13.jpc60002).

CARDS, Collaborative Atorvastatin Diabetes Study: Study not yet published. Info available at: www.theheart.org. (Accessed June 18, 2003). Written communication; Elizabeth Chebli, Pfizer US Medical Communications. July 21, 2003.

CARE, Cholesterol and Recurrent Events Trial: *N Engl J Med* 1996;335:1001–9; CCAIT, Canadian Coronary Atherosclerosis Intervention Trial: *Circulation* 1994;89:959–68. *Circulation* 1995; 92:2404–10.

FATS, Familial Atherosclerosis Treatment Study: *N Engl J Med* 1990;323:1289–98.

FLORIDA, Fluvastatin on Risk Diminishing after Acute Myocardial Infarction: [Abstract] *Circulation* 2000;102:2672d or www.acc.org/education/online/trials/aha00.

GREACE, GREek Atorvastatin and Coronary-heart-disease Evaluation study: *Curr Med Res Opin* 2002;18:220–8.

HATS, HDL Atherosclerosis Treatment Study: *N Engl J Med* 2001;345:1583–92.

HPS, Heart Protection Study: *Lancet* 2002;360:7–22. *Lancet* 2003;361:2005–16.

KAPS, Kuopio Atherosclerosis Prevention Study: *Circulation* 1995;92:1758–64.

LCAS, Lipoprotein and Coronary Atherosclerosis Study: *Am J Cardiol* 1997;80:278–86.

L-CAD, Lipid-Coronary Artery Disease Study: *Am J Cardiol* 2000;86:1293–8.

LIPID, Long-term Intervention with Pravastatin in Ischemic Disease: *N Engl J Med*1998;339:1349–57.

LIPS, *Lescol* Intervention Prevention Study: *JAMA* 2002;3215–22.

MAAS, Multicentre Anti-Atheroma Study: *Lancet* 1994;344:633–8.

MARS, Monitored Atherosclerosis Regression Study: *Ann Intern Med* 1993;119:969–76.

METEOR, Measuring Effects on intima media Thickness: an Evaluation Of Rosuvastatin: JAMA 2007; 297:1344–53.

MIRACL, Myocardial Ischemia Reduction with Aggressive Cholesterol Lowering: *JAMA* 2001;285:1711–8.

PLAC-I, Pravastatin Limitation of Atherosclerosis in the Coronary arteries (PLAC-I): *J Am Coll Cardiol* 1995;26:1133–9.

PLAC-II, Pravastatin Limitation of Atherosclerosis in the Carotid arteries. *Am J Cardiol* 1995;75:455–9.

PROSPER, Prevention of First Stroke: *Lancet* 2002;360:1623–30.

PROVE-IT, Pravastatin or Atorvastatin Evaluation and Infection Therapy: *N Engl J Med* 2004;350 (early release).

REGRESS, Regression Growth Evaluation Study: *Circulation* 1995;91:2528–40.

REVERSAL, Reversal of Atherosclerosis with Aggressive Lipid Lowering. *JAMA* 2004;291:1071–80.

SCAT, Simvastatin/Enalapril Coronary Atherosclerosis Trial: *Circulation* 2000;102:1748–54.

TREADMILL, Treatment of Peripheral Atherosclerotic Disease with Moderate or Intensive Lipid Lowering: Creager MA, et al [Abstract]. Presented at the 14th International Symposium on Drugs Affecting Lipid Metabolism, New York, September 9-13, 2001. Mohler E, et al. [Abstract]. Presented at: the 75th Scientific Sessions of the American Heart Association, Chicago, November 17–20, 2002.

WOSCOPS, West of Scotland Coronary Prevention Study: *N Engl J Med* 1995;333:1301–7.

[a] Based on United States product labeling and relevant studies. Canadian product information is given if it differs from US labeling.

[b] FDA-labeled indications. Evidence is level A for all studies except CARDS, FLORIDA, TREADMILL (which is level A/B) and GREACE and L-CAD (which are level B).

[c] In patients who have congestive heart disease or congestive heart disease risk-equivalent (diabetes, peripheral arterial disease, history of stroke or other cerebrovascular disease).

From Cholesterol-lowering agents. Pharmacist's Letter. Prescriber's Letter 2006;22(8):220802; with permission. Available at: www.prescribersletter.com. Accessed December 2007.

their use often requires some creativity and certainly a little extra time on the part of the health care provider. Statin-sensitive patients should be prescribed low doses of statins initially, because intolerance tends to be dose related, and the dosage titrated slowly [10,11]. The practitioner should not try to achieve these patients' target LDL level with the first dose.

Statin dosing typically is once daily, except for lovastatin, which can be taken twice daily. Table 2 outlines statins from the least to the most potent. In more sensitive patients, however, practitioners have used twice weekly or thrice weekly statin dosing successfully. Practitioners usually can find a statin dose that is tolerated by the patient.

At times, the statin dose that the patient tolerates does not achieve the patient's target LDL level. In that case, there are a few options to consider: adding ezetimibe, a resin, or prescription niacin (Niaspan). All these treatment options can help lower the LDL cholesterol [12]. Sometimes it is necessary to use a combination of these medications in conjunction with the statin to achieve the patient's target LDL level [1].

Adding ezetimibe or resin to any statin dose is a safe and effective way to lower LDL and avoid side effects from higher-dose statins [2]. It is well documented that doubling the statin dose lowers the LDL level by an additional 6%, but adding ezetimibe lowers the LDL level by 20% [13]. For statin-sensitive patients, adding ezetimibe to a smaller dose of statin is a viable option for combination therapy. Resins are another safe and effective option for combination therapy with a lower-dose statin. Dosing directions for resins are a little more complicated because of their tendency to reduce the absorption of other medications. With most resins (eg. cholestyramine or colestipol), the patient should be instructed to take other medications at least 1 hour before or 4 to 6 hours after taking the resin. Colesevelam (Welchol) is the newest resin available and has the best gastrointestinal tolerability [1,10]. It does not require any special dosing other than being taken with a meal and liquid, once daily or in divided doses. For truly statin-intolerant patients the only pharmacologic options for lowering LDL cholesterol may be ezetimibe or a resin, used as monotherapy or in combination [12].

Initiating and maintaining a patient on niacin treatment is another challenging issue for health care providers. Niacin actually improves all lipid parameters and is considered the drug of choice to raise high-density lipoprotein (HDL) cholesterol

effectively. It also has been shown to reduce the incidence of major coronary artery events [5,14].

Niacin has a long history of poor tolerability and patient noncompliance because of side effects. Various studies have reported niacin discontinuation rates ranging from 46% to 71% [14]. Niacin should not be prescribed without a fair amount of patient education.

Flushing, itching, and gastrointestinal issues tend to be the biggest tolerability issues that lead patients to discontinue the medication. Compliance rates can be improved significantly by using the sustained release form, Niaspan. Discussing why the medication is being prescribed, reviewing the side effects thoroughly, and educating the patients about the special dosing directions also can help compliance.

The flushing and itching that patients experience are not allergic reactions but are caused by the body's increased release of prostaglandin as the niacin is metabolized [5]. Patients should be prepared for the flushing or itching sensations they may experience before they receive samples or a prescription. They should be aware that everyone flushes or itches to some degree with this medication until their body gets used to the medication. It is wise for patients to believe they are supposed to flush; then, if they do not experience flushing or itching, they consider the absence of side effects a bonus. The health care provider should reassure patients that the flushing or itching is not cause for alarm and that these sensations resolve on their own, usually within 15 to 30 minutes. Occasionally the flush may last longer. These symptoms should not keep coming back throughout the night or into the next day. The subcutaneous redness the patient sees and feels is the result of the surface blood vessels dilating. Patients tend to have a positive response to this explanation, because they consider open or dilated blood vessels as a healthy condition and therefore are more willing to tolerate the symptoms.

Special dosing directions should be discussed and given to the patient. Niaspan should be started at a bedtime dose of 500 mg and titrated by 500 mg every 4 to 8 weeks to a maximum dose of 2000 mg/d. Titration should not be rushed, especially if the patient is having problems with tolerability. With each titration patients should be reminded to expect an increased flush until they are accustomed to the higher dose [14].

A few tips can help make patients more comfortable while they get used to the effects of Niaspan. If the patient is able to take an aspirin or a nonsteroidal antiinflammatory drug, they should do so 30 minutes before taking Niaspan. This pretreatment reduces the flushing and itching by inhibiting the formation of prostaglandin, caused by the Niaspan [15]. Niaspan always should be taken with a low-fat or fat-free snack. Fatty snacks, such as peanut-butter crackers, tend to increase the flushing sensation. Hot beverages, spicy foods, and alcohol also increase the flushing sensation. For better tolerability, the patient should be reminded not to cut or crush the tablets [2]. Pharmaceutical companies offer tear-off sheets that list these directions and sheets that explain what the flush feels like.

If the patient calls the health care provider complaining of intolerable flushing or itching, one should confirm that the patient is following all the dosing directions. Often these directions are not being followed. A few additional tips can be suggested if needed. One is taking Niaspan at supper time. One should stress again that the meal should be low in fat. If the flush is intolerable, benadryl can be used with Niaspan for a short time until the patient can become accustomed to the Niaspan. If the complaints follow a recent titration of Niaspan, one could consider reducing the Niaspan dose for a few more weeks before titrating.

When prescribing Niaspan to raise HDL cholesterol, one should notify the patient that other drug options are limited. Educating patients and building their confidence about taking Niaspan before it is prescribed are worth the investment of time by the health care provider.

Summary

Trying to manage cholesterol levels in difficult-to-treat patients is one of the many challenges health care providers face. Finding an acceptable treatment option can require diligent work on the part of the health care provider and the patient. The suggestions provided in this article will give the practitioner some options that might increase patient compliance when starting a treatment plan for hyperlipidemia.

References

[1] Toth PP. Expert commentary: gastrointestinally active lipid-lowering drug safety. Am J Cardiol 2007; 99:56–8.

[2] Stone NJ, Blum CB. Management of lipids in clinical practice. 6th edition. New York: Professional Communications, Inc.; 2006. p. 300–1.

[3] Armitage J. The safety of stains in clinical practice review. Lancet 2007;370:1781–90.

[4] Grundy SM. The issue of statin safety. Where do we stand? Circulation 2005;111:3016–9.

[5] Stone NJ. Combination therapy lowering LDL. Emerging paradigms in lipid care. In: Proceedings from the 2003 Southeast Lipid Association Annual Scientific Forum. Jacksonville (FL): National Lipid Association; 2004. p. 28–32.

[6] Lopes-Virella M, Huang Y. Insights on plaque vulnerability and acute coronary syndromes. The Lipid Spin 2006;4:1–9.

[7] Toth PP. Statins and myopathy. The Lipid Spin 2007;4:11–23.

[8] Graham DJ, Staffa JA, Shatin D, et al. Incidence of hospitalized rhabdomyolysis in patients treated with lipid-lowering drugs. JAMA 2004;292:2585–90.

[9] Vasudevan AR, Hamirani YS, Jones PH. Safety of statins: effects on muscle and the liver. Cleve Clin J Med 2005;72:990–1000.

[10] Jacobson TA, Armani A, McKenney JM, et al. Safety considerations with gastrointestinally active lipid lowering drugs. Am J Cardiol 2007;99:46–55.

[11] Statin vs. statin LDL lowering at various doses. Available at: www.prescribersletter.com. Accessed December 2007.

[12] Toth PP. Colesevelam for the management of dyslipidemia. The Lipid Spin 2006;4:14.

[13] Toth PP. Ezetimide: mechanism of action and effects on serum lipoproteins. The Lipid Spin 2005;3:11–2.

[14] Gotto A, Pownall H. Manual of lipid disorders reducing the risk for coronary artery disease. New York: Lippincott Williams & Wilkins; 2003. p. 299–354.

[15] Stern RH. The role of nicotinic acid metabolites in flushing and hepatotoxicity. J Clin Lipidol 2007;1: 191–3.

CRITICAL CARE
NURSING CLINICS
OF NORTH AMERICA

Crit Care Nurs Clin N Am 20 (2008) 297–304

Cardiovascular Disease Prevention in Women: The Role of the Nurse Practitioner in Primary Care

Roberta E. Hoebeke, RN, PhD, FNP-BC

College of Nursing and Health Professions, University of Southern Indiana, 8600 University Boulevard,
Evansville, IN 47712, USA

Cardiovascular disease in women

Cardiovascular disease (CVD) is the most prevalent health problem in the United States and includes the following health conditions: high blood pressure, coronary heart disease (including myocardial infarction and angina pectoris), heart failure, and stroke. The most recent prevalence data from 2005 national surveys indicated that approximately 80,700,000 Americans have CVD. Of these, 42,700,000 are women, and 37,900,000 are men [1].

Mortality

For every year since 1900, except for 1918, CVD has been the primary cause of death in the United States [1]. CVD is the number one cause of death among women in the United States and throughout the world. CVD causes 8.6 million deaths per year worldwide among women. One third of all women's deaths worldwide are attributed to CVD [2]. More women than men die each year from CVD in the United States. Of the almost 1 million deaths caused by CVD in the United States in 2004, 459,096 (52.8%) were women, and 410,628 (47.2%) were men. In that year more women died from CVD than from cancer, chronic lower respiratory disease, accidents, diabetes, and Alzheimer's combined [1]. During the past 25 years there has been a trend of decreasing CVD mortality trend for men, and more women than men have died of CVD every year since 1984 [1].

Cost

In 2008 it is estimated that CVD morbidity and mortality will cost the United States economy $448.5 billion in health care expenditures and lost productivity [1]. Tracking the prevalence of risk factors for CVD, the Centers for Disease Control and Prevention (CDC) data from the 2003 Behavioral Risk Factor Surveillance System showed that between 1990 and 2000 young women age 18 to 24 years had the highest rates of several risk factors associated with developing CVD: smoking, large increases in obesity, high levels of sedentary behavior, and low fruit and vegetable intake [1]. These risk factors will translate into millions more cases of CVD in women during the ensuing decades, increasing the personal and economic burden of CVD. Currently, the lifetime risk of a 40-year-old woman in the United States for developing CVD is more than one in two, so prevention, risk assessment, and addressing risk factors for CVD are crucial for women's health [1]. Most CVD in women is preventable, and decreasing the death rate by just 2% over a 10-year period would prevent 36 million deaths [3].

Awareness

Historically, women have perceived their risk for developing CVD to be low, falsely assuming that heart disease is mainly a disease of men. Surveys conducted by the American Heart Association (AHA) to assess women's awareness, perceptions, and knowledge of CVD found that in 1997 only 7% of women believed heart disease was a major threat to their health [4]. In 2003 awareness had increased only to 13%, but in 2006 the percentage of women who were aware

E-mail address: rhoebeke@usi.edu

that heart disease was a leading cause of death among women had risen to 57% [1,4]. Awareness is lower among African American and Hispanic women than in white women. Historically, physicians have believed that women have a lower risk of heart disease than men, and this misperception has been reflected in practice with fewer recommendations regarding CVD preventive measures made to women patients than to men with similar risk profiles [4,5]. In a study conducted by the AHA, one in five women stated her health care provider did not explain clearly how she could improve her CVD risk status, and 25% said the health care provider did not tell them that heart health was important [6].

Guidelines for prevention of cardiovascular disease in women

Previously, studies were lacking with sufficient numbers of women to make CVD prevention recommendations for women. Beginning in 1999, the AHA published "A Guide to Preventive Cardiology in Women," which was a scientific statement based on data from a 1997 review of the literature that reported CVD occurrence, risk factors, and their management in women [7]. Since 2004, evidence-based guidelines for the prevention of CVD in women based on clinical trial data from women have been developed and published [8]. The 2007 update of these evidence-based guidelines provides the most recent recommendations for CVD prevention in women age 20 years and older, with specific contraindications for women who are pregnant or wish to become pregnant [9]. By following these guidelines and using them in clinical practice, nurse practitioners (NPs) in primary care settings are in a prime position to provide CVD risk assessment and prevention strategies to women across the lifespan.

Assessment of risk factors for cardiovascular disease

The AHA 2007 update guidelines for prevention of CVD in women emphasize that the first step is to assess a woman's risk factors for CVD and then to classify her level of risk as high risk, at risk, or optimal risk (Box 1) [9]. To determine CVD risk, the NP elicits the past medical and family history (including a family history of CVD and familial/genetic conditions such as hypercholesterolemia) and lifestyle and health habits, calculates the Framingham risk score,

---

Box 1. Classification of the risk of cardiovascular disease (CVD) in women

High risk
Established coronary heart disease
Cerebrovascular disease
Peripheral arterial disease
Abdominal aortic aneurysm
End-stage or chronic renal disease
10-Year Framingham global risk greater than 20%[a]
Diabetes mellitus

At risk
One or more major risk factors for CVD, including
- Cigarette smoking
- Poor diet
- Physical inactivity
- Obesity, especially central adiposity
- Family history of premature CVD (CVD at age < 55 years of age in a male relative or < 65 years of age in a female relative)
- Hypertension
- Dyslipidemia
Evidence of subclinical vascular disease (eg, coronary calcification)
Metabolic syndrome
Poor exercise capacity on treadmill test and/or abnormal heart rate recovery after stopping exercise

Optimal risk
Framingham global risk less than 10% and a healthful lifestyle, with no risk factors.

---

[a] Or at high risk on the basis of another population-adapted tool used to assess global risk.
Adapted from American Heart Association. Evidence-based guidelines for cardiovascular disease prevention in women: 2007 update. Circulation 2007;115:1481–501; with permission.

---

and conducts a review of systems for symptoms of CVD. Women who have CVD should be screened for depression. The NP performs a physical examination and obtains blood pressure, waist measurement, and body mass index measurements. Laboratory values, including a fasting lipid profile and glucose level, are obtained. NPs in primary care settings can perform all these tasks effectively.

Earlier guidelines for CVD assessment of women used a more detailed classification system of high risk, intermediate risk, lower risk, and optimal risk [8]. Central to determining risk classification and making preventive recommendations for women under the 2004 guidelines was the Framingham 10-year global risk score [10]. To calculate risk level, the Framingham score uses age, gender, total cholesterol and high-density lipoprotein (HDL) cholesterol values, systolic blood pressure, and smoking status to tally points. The point total is used to estimate the 10-year risk of coronary heart disease, expressed as a percentage.

Recent studies suggest the Framingham tool has some limitations for risk stratification in women. New evidence finds that a woman's risk can be over- or underestimated depending on her ethnicity, and many women who were categorized as low risk had documented subclinical disease. The Framingham criteria still are used to guide the health care provider in prescribing lipid therapy. For risk classification, the Framingham tool is reliable in identifying women at high risk (eg, > 20%), but a lower score does not ensure a lower risk in women. Also, the Framingham tool focuses on short-term (10-year) absolute risk rather than lifetime risk. Because the average lifetime risk for CVD in women is one in two, which is very high, it is of paramount importance to apply prevention strategies to all women and to emphasize a heart-healthy lifestyle [11].

The major changes from the 2004 guidelines that are reflected in the AHA 2007 update guidelines include a greater emphasis on lifetime risk instead of the short-term 10-year absolute risk estimated by the Framingham score and modification of the risk categories. The roles of screening technologies such as high-sensitivity C-reactive protein and coronary calcium scoring in CVD risk stratification have not been determined in the AHA 2007 guidelines update, because more research studies are needed to determine their benefit. Similarly, further studies are needed to explore unique risks during pregnancy (eg, history of pre-eclampsia) and their relationship to the lifetime risk of CVD.

Recommendations for clinical prevention of cardiovascular disease

The next step in applying the AHA 2007 update guidelines is to implement the evidence-based CVD prevention recommendations for women. These clinical recommendations to lower women's CVD risk factors are divided into three categories [9]:

- Lifestyle interventions
- Major risk factor interventions
- Preventive drug interventions

Interventions that are not useful or effective or that may be harmful are discussed also. Each recommendation and the role of the NP in primary care are described in the following sections. To assist the NP in implementing these clinical recommendations, an algorithm is provided in Fig. 1.

Lifestyle interventions

Health-promotion counseling on heart-healthy lifestyle interventions, including smoking cessation, regular physical activity, healthy diet, and weight maintenance, is important for all women, independent of their risk level. Barriers to health care providers counseling patients about lifestyle changes can include lack of time during the patient visit, lack of confidence about how to address these changes, and/or the perception that the patient will not be able to make the needed changes. Approaches such as motivational interviewing have demonstrated that encouraging patient participation in the decision-making process and taking an encouraging/affirming rather than a judgmental or lecturing approach is effective in motivating patients to take an active part in lifestyle modification [12]. This approach incorporates active listening, and the patients and provider work collaboratively to set goals and develop a plan to help patients achieve healthy lifestyle outcomes. This approach empowers women to make the decision to change their lifestyle behaviors and to follow through on their decisions with the confidence and motivation to succeed.

Cigarette smoking

Smoking is a major risk factor for CVD, and women who smoke double their risk of stroke [2]. The NP should encourage women to stop smoking. NPs should ask about smoking at every primary care visit. NPs can offer smoking cessation assistance to help women achieve their goal to stop smoking by providing behavioral counseling or referral to smoking cessation programs in conjunction with pharmacotherapy. NPs also should counsel women to avoid second-hand smoke. Exposure to second-hand smoke increases a woman's risk of dying from heart disease by 15% [2].

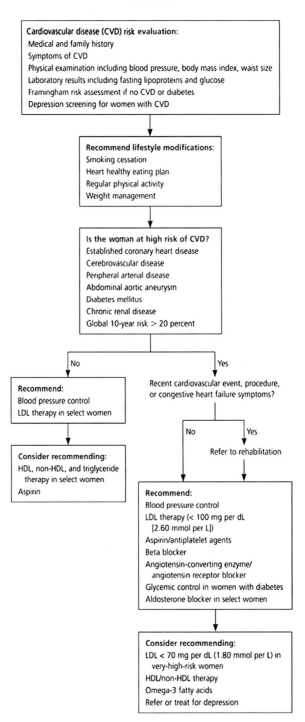

Fig. 1. Preventing cardiovascular disease in women. CVD, cardiovascular disease; HDL, high-density lipoprotein; LDL, low-density lipoprotein. *Adapted from* American Heart Association. Evidence-based guidelines for cardiovascular disease prevention in women: 2007 update. Circulation 2007;115:1481–501; with permission.

Physical activity

Women who accumulate less than 1 hour per week of physical activity increase their risk of developing CVD by 1.58 times compared with women who engage in physical activity more than 3 hours per week [2]. NPs should urge all women to get at least 30 minutes of brisk walking or other moderate-intensity physical activity on most days and preferably every day. The NP can help women plan for fitting more physical activity into their day and ask at each visit how these strategies are working. For women who need to lose weight or maintain their weight loss, NPs should recommend 60 to 90 minutes of moderate-intensity physical activity on most, and preferably all, days.

Dietary intake

The NP should encourage healthful eating patterns, including whole grains, high-fiber foods, a variety of fruits and vegetables, low-fat or non-fat dairy, and legumes and lean sources of protein with low saturated fat content. Saturated fat intake should be less than 10% of total calories (< 7% for high-risk women), trans-fat should be avoided as much as possible and should comprise less than 1% of daily calories, and cholesterol should be less than 300 mg/day (< 200 mg in women at high risk). Eating fish, especially oily fish high in omega-3 fatty acids such as salmon, should be encouraged twice a week. Pregnant or lactating women are an exception: they should avoid eating fish that could be high in mercury (eg, mackerel, tilefish, swordfish, or shark). These women are encouraged to eat up to 12 ounces per week of other varieties of fish and shellfish that are deemed low in mercury by the Environmental Protection Agency and the US Food and Drug Administration. Sodium should be limited to about 1 teaspoon per day (< 2.3 g). Alcohol can be consumed in moderation but should be limited to no more than one 5-ounce glass of wine per day, or one 12-ounce beer, or one 1.5-ounce shot of liquor per day. The NP can provide written dietary materials and basic diet counseling as part of the primary care visit. The NP may refer women at higher risk to a dietician or nutritionist for professional guidance on a prescribed therapeutic diet.

Weight maintenance

The risk of an obese woman's dying of CVD is 1.45 that of healthy woman of normal weight [2]. Height and weight should be measured in the primary care setting to determine body mass index, and waist circumference should be measured. Women should be encouraged to lose weight if needed and to maintain a healthy body mass index between 18.5 and 24.9 and a waist circumference less than 35 inches. The NP can discuss the relationship between body mass index and waist circumference and CVD risk with the patient. Using motivational interviewing techniques, the NP can help women set goals and implement strategies to achieve a proper balance of physical activity and calorie intake and can recommend formal behavioral weight-loss programs as appropriate.

Omega-3 fatty acids

The NP may consider recommending that high-risk women who have high triglyceride levels or heart disease take omega-3 fatty acid supplements as an adjunct to a heart-healthy diet. The AHA 2007 update guidelines recommend that women who have heart disease take 850 mg to 1000 mg of eicosapentaenoic acid and docosahexaenoic acid in capsule form and that women who have high triglyceride levels take higher doses of 2 to 4 g/d.

Depression

The weight of the evidence is in favor of interventions to screen for and treat depression in women at high risk for CVD. Depression affects more women than men, and depression is a barrier to engaging in healthy lifestyle behaviors. Women who are treated for depression may have a reduced risk of adverse outcomes from heart disease [13]. The NP should use a valid and reliable depression tool to screen high-risk women who have CVD for depression. If depression is identified, the NP must take measures to treat it within the scope of advanced practice nursing and refer as appropriate.

Rehabilitation

For women who have had a recent coronary intervention, acute coronary syndrome, a recent cerebrovascular accident, new-onset or chronic angina, peripheral arterial disease, or heart failure symptoms, the NP should discuss and offer referral to a comprehensive cardiac risk-reduction program. Depending on the nature of the problem, referral could be to a cardiac rehabilitation program, a stroke rehabilitation program, or an in-home or community-based physician-guided exercise-training program.

Major risk factor interventions

In addition to lifestyle interventions, the AHA 2007 update guidelines recommend blood pressure control and management of hyperlipidemia for women who are at risk and for women at high risk. Treatments may vary depending on whether women have multiple risk factors, including diabetes, or if they have contraindications to certain blood pressure– or lipid-lowering medications.

Blood pressure

The NP should encourage maintenance of an optimal blood pressure ($<$ 120/80 mm Hg) through lifestyle approaches (eg, a diet rich in fruits and vegetables with low-fat dairy products and moderate alcohol and low sodium intake). Physical activity and healthy weight control and maintenance also should be emphasized. The NP needs to prescribe pharmacotherapy to prevent target organ damage in women whose blood pressure is 140/90 mm Hg or higher, or even at lower pressure ($\geq$ 130/80 mm Hg) in women who have chronic renal disease or diabetes. Thiazide diuretics should be considered first-line therapy for most women unless they are contraindicated or there are compelling reasons to use other agents specific to certain conditions. For women at high risk of CVD, beta-blockers alone or in combination with angiotensin-converting enzyme (ACE) inhibitors or angiotensin-receptor blockers (ARBs) are recommended as initial treatment, with thiazide diuretics added as needed to achieve optimal blood pressure goals.

Lipids

The NP also should encourage lifestyle approaches to help women achieve and maintain optimal lipid levels. According to the AHA 2007 update guidelines, optimal low-density lipoprotein (LDL) cholesterol levels should be less than 100 mg/dL, and HDL cholesterol levels should be greater than 50 mg/dL for women. Optimal triglyceride levels are less than 150 mg/dL, and non-HDL cholesterol value (the total cholesterol minus HDL cholesterol) should be less than 130 mg/dL. The NP should initiate LDL cholesterol–lowering therapy for any woman, regardless of risk factors, who has an LDL cholesterol level of 190 mg/dL or greater on lifestyle therapy alone. The NP should initiate LDL cholesterol–lowering therapy if the LDL cholesterol is 160 mg/dL or higher with lifestyle therapy alone and multiple risk factors are present, even if the 10-year Framingham absolute risk is less than 10%. As a woman's risk status increases (eg, when multiple risk factors are present, and the 10-year Framingham absolute risk is 10%–20%), the NP should implement LDL cholesterol–lowering therapy if the LDL cholesterol is 130 mg/dL or higher.

If women have high-risk conditions or elevated LDL cholesterol levels, the NP should implement LDL cholesterol–lowering therapy with statins, unless contraindicated, to achieve an LDL cholesterol level of less than 100 mg/dL concomitantly with lifestyle approaches including a very low dietary intake of saturated fat ($<$ 7%), trans-fat ($<$ 1%) and daily cholesterol intake of less than 200 mg/day. For women at very high risk (eg, women who have diabetes and coronary heart disease), the target LDL cholesterol level is less than 70 mg/dL. Fibric acid or niacin therapy should be implemented for women in this population who have low HDL cholesterol levels and high non-HDL cholesterol levels .

Diabetes

The risk of coronary death is 3.5 higher for premenopausal women who have type 2 diabetes than for nondiabetic premenopausal women. The risk of CVD death of a woman who has diabetes is significantly higher than that of a man who has diabetes [2]. Tight control of diabetes leads to more favorable outcomes and fewer CVD-related events compared with less optimal glucose control. The NP should institute lifestyle approaches and pharmacotherapy to achieve a target hemoglobin A_{1C} level of less than 7%, if this level can be achieved without significant hypoglycemia.

Preventive drug interventions

Aspirin

The NP should offer aspirin therapy at 75 mg to 325 mg/d to all women in the high-risk category, unless they are allergic or have other contraindications. If aspirin cannot be tolerated, clopidogrel (Plavix) can be substituted. Healthy women younger than age 65 years should not use aspirin routinely to prevent myocardial infarction, however. The NP can recommend aspirin therapy of 81 mg/d or 100 mg every other day to women 65 years and older to prevent ischemic stroke and myocardial infarction, as long as blood pressure is controlled. According to the AHA 2007 update guidelines, the benefits of this therapy are likely to outweigh the risks of potential gastrointestinal bleeding and hemorrhagic stroke. These recommendations also apply to women younger than

65 years when the benefits of preventing ischemic stroke outweigh the risks of the aspirin therapy.

Beta-blockers

In accordance with the AHA 2007 update guidelines, beta-blockers should be used indefinitely, unless contraindicated, by all women who have chronic ischemic syndromes, left ventricular dysfunction with or without heart failure symptoms, and after a myocardial infarction.

Angiotensin-converting enzyme inhibitors/ angiotensin-receptor blockers

The NP should consider using ACE-inhibitors, unless contraindicated, in high-risk women (eg, women who have diabetes, women who have had a myocardial infarction, or women in heart failure or with a left ventricular ejection fraction of 40% or less). If women are intolerant of ACE inhibitors, ARBs should be considered instead. These recommendations are contraindicated in women who are pregnant or who wish to become pregnant.

Aldosterone blockade

The NP should consider using aldosterone blockade for women who have had a myocardial infarction, who are diabetic (but who do not have significant renal dysfunction or hyperkalemia), or who have heart failure and are already taking therapeutic doses of a beta-blocker and an ACE inhibitor.

Interventions that are not useful/effective and may be harmful

The AHA 2007 update guidelines revised the earlier 2004 guidelines to reflect current evidence from recently published randomized trials related to the use of menopausal therapy, antioxidant supplements, folic acid, and aspirin [9].

Menopausal therapy

The NP should not prescribe hormone therapy, whether combined estrogen plus progestin or other menopausal hormone therapy, or selective estrogen-receptor modulator therapy for primary or secondary prevention of CVD or myocardial infarction in postmenopausal women.

Antioxidant supplements

Based on current evidence, the NP should not recommend antioxidant supplements such as vitamins C, E, or beta-carotene for primary or secondary prevention of CVD or myocardial infarction in women.

Folic acid

Under the 2004 guidelines, folic acid supplements were considered an adjunct to therapy for women at high risk of CVD if they had higher-than-normal homocysteine levels [8]. The AHA 2007 update guidelines report that current evidence does not support the use of folic acid supplements, with or without vitamin B_6 and B_{12}, for primary or secondary prevention of CVD or myocardial infarction in women. Women of childbearing age are an exception: the NP should recommend that these women take folic acid supplements to prevent neural tube defects.

Aspirin in women younger than 65 years

Based on findings from the Women's Health Initiative study, the risks of myocardial infarction in women are not reduced by aspirin use except for women older than 65 years. This finding was in contrast to the effects of aspirin for primary prevention of CVD in men. Therefore, the NP should not routinely recommend aspirin to prevent heart attack in women younger than 65 years. The overall risks of ischemic stroke were decreased by 24% in the population younger than 65 years, but significant bleeding complications rose by 40% in those taking aspirin [14].

Summary

NPs frequently see women in the primary care setting for health-promotion/wellness visits as well as for treatment of acute, episodic illnesses and management of chronic disease. NPs are in a prime position to offer CVD lifestyle intervention counseling and to implement risk-factor reduction and preventive pharmacotherapy interventions to women within the context of these visits. Research has demonstrated consistently that the quality of care and patients' satisfaction with care provided by NPs is high, and that primary care outcomes of patients managed by NPs are comparable to those of patients managed by physicians [15]. As the physician shortage in primary care deepens, NPs will be first-line health care providers for millions of women. The NP can offer a first line of defense against the development of CVD in women by consistently putting into practice the approaches outlined in the AHA 2007 update guidelines.

References

[1] Rosamond W, Flegal K, Furie K, et al. for the American Heart Association Statistics Committee and Stroke Statistics Subcommittee. Heart disease and stroke statistics—2008 update: a report from the American Heart Association Statistics Committee and Stroke Statistics subcommittee. Circulation 2008;117(4):e25–146.

[2] World Heart Federation. Women. Available at: http://www.worldheartfederation.org/press/factsfigures/women/print.html? Accessed January 21, 2008.

[3] Strong K, Mathers C, Leeder S, et al. Preventing chronic diseases: how many lives can we save? Lancet 2005;366(9496):1578–82.

[4] Mosca L, Ferris A, Fabunmi R, et al. Tracking women's awareness of heart disease: an American Heart Association national study. Circulation 2004;109(5):573–9.

[5] Mosca L, Linfante AH, Benjamin EJ, et al. National study of physician awareness and adherence to cardiovascular disease prevention guidelines. Circulation 2005;111(4):499–510.

[6] Mosca L, Mochari H, Christian AH, et al. National study of women's awareness, preventive action, and barriers to cardiovascular health. Circulation 2006; 113(4):525–34.

[7] Mosca L, Grundy SM, Judelson D, et al. Guide to preventive cardiology for women: AHA/ACC scientific statement consensus panel statement. Circulation 1999;99(18):2480–4.

[8] Mosca L, Appel LJ, Benjamin EJ, et al, for the American Heart Association. Evidence-based guidelines for cardiovascular disease prevention in women. Circulation 2004;109(5):672–93.

[9] Mosca L, Banka CL, Benjamin EJ, et al, for the Expert Panel/Writing Group. Evidence-based guidelines for cardiovascular disease prevention in women: 2007 update. Circulation 2007;115(11):1481–501.

[10] National Cholesterol Education Program (NCEP) Expert Panel on Detection, Evaluation, and Treatment of High Blood Cholesterol in Adults (Adult Treatment Panel III). Third report of the National Cholesterol Education Program (NCEP) Expert Panel on Detection, Evaluation, and Treatment of High Blood Cholesterol in Adults (Adult Treatment Panel III) final report. Circulation 2002;106(25):3143–421.

[11] Sibley C, Blumenthal RS, Bairey Merz CN, et al. Limitations of current cardiovascular disease risk assessment strategies in women. J Womens Health (Larchmt) 2006;15(1):54–6.

[12] Miller WR, Rollnick S. Motivational interviewing: preparing people for change. 2nd edition. New York: Guilford Press; 2002.

[13] Taylor CB, Youngblood ME, Catellier D, et al. Effects of antidepressant medication on morbidity and mortality in depressed patients after myocardial infarction. Arch Gen Psychiatry 2005;62(7):792–8.

[14] Ridker PM, Cook NR, Lee IM, et al. A randomized trial of low-dose aspirin in the primary prevention of cardiovascular disease in women. N Engl J Med 2005;352(13):1293–304.

[15] Lenz ER, Mundinger MO, Kane RL, et al. Primary care outcomes in patients treated by nurse practitioners or physicians: two-year follow-up. Med Care Res Rev 2004;61(3):332–51.

ELSEVIER
SAUNDERS

Crit Care Nurs Clin N Am 20 (2008) 305–310

CRITICAL CARE
NURSING CLINICS
OF NORTH AMERICA

Managing Hypertension in Women

Mary Jane Swartz, RN, MSN, ACNS-BC

8211 Peach Blossom Lane, Evansville, IN 47715, USA

Hypertension has been classified for several years as a "silent killer" because of the lack of associated symptoms. However, hypertension is linked to the development of target organ disease, which leads to cardiovascular and renal disease. Stroke and heart disease rank high in the leading causes of death in the United States and are major contributions to the financial and societal costs in health care. Hypertension is listed as the most common primary diagnosis in America. Therefore, controlling hypertension can be an important factor to reducing the incidence of these prevalent public health concerns.

This article discusses the findings outlined in The Seventh Report of the Joint National Committee on Prevention, Detection, Evaluation, and Treatment of High Blood Pressure (JNC 7) (www.nhlbi.hih.gov) [1]. Using evidence-based research, JNC 7 outlines a comprehensive approach to the challenges hypertension present for health care providers and patients. This article highlights the issues of hypertension in women. Studies suggest that age plays a major role in the development of hypertension throughout the life cycle. Women have lower systolic blood pressure during the early adulthood compared to men; whereas, at the age of fifty the likelihood of hypertension increase more for women versus men. During one's lifetime, women have a 86–90 percent chance of developing hypertension versus 81–83 percent risk for men. Therefore, prevention or control of hypertension is important for women's health.

What is high blood pressure?

In 2004, JNC 7 introduced a new classification system. The system was refined from the one published in the Sixth Report in 1997. The prehypertension stage was added to identify people for whom early interventions may delay or eliminate the diagnosis of hypertension. Recently gathered evidence supports controlling systolic blood pressure (SBP), which has a greater impact on cardiovascular disease. Blood pressure changes with age; the rise in SBP will continue until around 50 years of age and then level off. Because diastolic blood pressure seems to rise before 50 years of age, either alone or paired with systolic hypertension, diastolic hypertension is a greater cardiovascular risk factor, whereas attention should be directed to SBP after age 50 (Table 1).

What are keys to prevention?

Several factors play key roles in the risk for developing high blood pressure. Age seems to play a key role in the rise of SBP. After 50 years age, women have a higher incidence of developing high blood pressure than men. After 60 years of age, women have an equal or greater tendency to develop high blood pressure compared with men. Other health practices that contribute to blood pressure elevation include body weight over ideal, physical inactivity, poor intake of fruits and vegetables, overconsumption of dietary sodium, and excessive alcohol intake.

Several programs have been developed to alert the public about the dangers of hypertension and its effects. Healthy People 2010 is an initiative to disseminate information to diverse community groups on the risks and dangers of hypertension [2]. The American Heart Association created the Go Red for Women campaign to inform women that heart disease linked to hypertension is the number one killer of women [3]. This campaign uses the color red to give women information related to risk factor reduction, daily exercise, and

E-mail address: mswartz3@usi.edu

0899-5885/08/$ - see front matter © 2008 Elsevier Inc. All rights reserved.
doi:10.1016/j.ccell.2008.03.011

Table 1
Classification system from the seventh report of the joint
national committee on prevention, detection, and evaluation, and treatment of high blood pressure (JNC 7)

Systolic/diastolic blood pressure	JNC 7 category
<120/80	Normal
120–129/80/84	Prehypertension
130–139/85–89	Hypertension
140–159/90–99	Stage 1
160–179/100–09	Stage 2
>180/110	

Data from U.S. Department of Health and Human
Services; National Institutes of Health; National
Heart, Lung, and Blood Institute. The Seventh Report
of the Joint National Committee on Prevention, Detection, Evaluation, and Treatment of High Blood Pressure (JNC 7). Available at: http://www.nhlbi.nih.gov/
guidelines/hypertension/. Accessed April 15, 2008.

healthy eating. In addition, it promotes a program
called "know your numbers," which encourages
women to know and understand the heart-healthy
figures for total cholesterol, bad cholesterol
(low-density lipoprotein), good cholesterol (high-
density lipoprotein), triglycerides, blood pressure,
fasting glucose, body mass index, waist circumference, and exercise time.

Detection of high blood pressure

Discussion on the detection of hypertension
would be incomplete without emphasizing the
guidelines for accurate blood pressure
measurement:

- Sphygmomanometers should be inspected
  regularly.
- Before auscultation, individuals should be in
  a sitting position for at least 5 minutes with
  feet on the floor and the arm supported at
  the level of the heart.
- Auscultation is preferred for automatic
  detection.
- Patients should avoid exercise, smoking, and
  caffeine for at least 30 minutes before
  auscultation.
- An appropriately sized cuff must be used for
  accuracy.
- Operators should be skilled at identifying the
  Korotkoff sounds to differentiate systolic and
  diastole blood pressure.

Ambulatory blood pressure monitoring and
self-measurement are valuable in assessing blood

pressure during daily activities. These practices
are helpful for patients who have suspected white-
coat hypertension, and for regular monitoring in
those who are undergoing hypertensive medication regimes.

Findings of the National Health and Nutrition Examination Survey III showed that women
are more aware than men of having hypertension, and are more likely to visit the physician
regularly, which can assist in detection and
treatment.

Furthermore, health care provides should evaluate patients. This examination should include the
following:

- Determination of family or lifestyle risk
  factors
- Ruling out of identifiable causes of hypertension, such as drug-induced chronic kidney disease, sleep apnea, thyroid or parathyroid
  disease, and Cushing's syndrome
- Examination of the optic fundi
- Height and weight/body mass index
- Auscultation of heart and lungs
- Auscultation for carotid, abdominal, and
  femoral bruits
- Detection of elevated heart rate, which may
  suggest cardiovascular disease in absence of
  other risk factors

As part of the screening process or before the
start of an antihypertensive regimen, routine
laboratory tests are recommended. These tests
include 12-lead ECG, urinalysis, blood glucose,
hematocrit, serum potassium, serum calcium,
creatinine, and lipoprotein profile. The high-
sensitivity C-reactive protein (HS-CRP), which
is a marker of inflammation, may be elevated in
women with a higher risk for a cardiovascular
event. An elevation in homocysteine has been
linked to higher risk for cardiovascular damage
but not as closely as elevations in HS-CRP. If an
underlying cause of the hypertension is suspected
or blood pressure does not respond to antihypertensive agents, more intensive diagnostic tests
may be necessary.

The JNC 7 recommends basing follow-up
on initial blood pressure measurements for
adults who do not have acute end organ damage
(Table 2).

The goal of antihypertensive treatment as
outlined in JNC 7 is to reduce the morbidity and
mortality from the target organ damage related to
cardiovascular and renal systems.

Table 2
Follow-up recommendations based on initial blood pressure measurements for adults who have no acute end organ damage

Initial blood pressure	Follow-up recommendation
Optimal <120/80	Recheck in 2 years
Prehypertension Normal = 120–129/80–84 Borderline = 130–139/ 85–89	Recheck in 1 year
Stage 1 hypertension 140–159/90–99	Confirm within 2 months
Stage 2 hypertension 160–179/100–109 Stage 3 hypertension >180/110	Evaluate or refer to source of care within 1 month; For those who have higher pressures, evaluate and treat immediately or within 1 wk, depending on clinical situation and complications.

The first step in treating hypertension

Lifestyle modifications remain the initial and cornerstone approach to preventing and treating high blood pressure (Fig. 1). These modifications seem to have a higher gain for women than men. Adopting two or more of these modifications can have a strong impact on delaying the hypertension, augmenting the effectiveness of drug therapy, and reducing the risk on target organs.

The principles of lifestyle modifications are as follows:

- Achieve ideal weight; weight loss of at least 10 lb can affect blood pressure
- Adhere to the DASH (dietary approaches to stop hypertension) eating plan to help reduce cholesterol and total fat [4]
- Maintain a diet high in fruits and vegetables
- Reduce dietary intake of sodium to less than 2.4 g daily
- Include low-fat diary products in diet
- Engage in regular aerobic physical activity at least 30 minutes daily or most days of the week; finding ways to include physical activity in the daily routines are recommended, such as using the stairs rather than the elevator or taking a brisk walk at lunch
- Stop smoking
- Limit alcohol intake to less than 1 oz/d; this amount equals two drinks per day for a man and one drink daily for a woman.

Pharmacologic choices for treating hypertension

Several medications involve many drug classes available to treat hypertension. Based on several clinical trials, more than two thirds of patients who have hypertension will require two or more antihypertensive medications from the different drug classes to achieve the goal blood pressure. The first medication used to treat hypertension should be a diuretic, which is generally well tolerated. The cost of the medication, timing of doses, and use of combination medications should be considered.

Compliance with medication scheduling remains a concern for patients taking medication for hypertension with no symptoms. Health care providers must educate patients on the treatment plan for hypertension, which includes a multifaceted approach involving lifestyle modifications, stress management, and compliance with drug therapy. For patients who do not adhere to the treatment plan, health care providers must listen to their concerns. Factors identified as reasons for noncompliance include cost, inadequate instructions, lack of patient involvement in the treatment plan, side effects of medication, and inconvenient dosing.

Box 1 lists the classes of drugs, provides a brief description, and describes actions [5].

Based on clinical trials, JNC 7 provides guidelines for individual drug classes according to patient high-risk conditions that are a direct result of target organ damage, which are compelling indications for certain antihypertensive medications. Box 2 outlines the compelling indication and recommended drug class.

After an antihypertensive medication is initiated, patients should be monitored monthly until the target blood pressure is obtained. After the goal is reached, visits can occur every 3 to 6 months. Yearly laboratory testing should include serum potassium and creatinine.

Best drug classifications for women

Studies indicate that the different classifications of antihypertensive drugs can produce the same effect in women and men. Gender differences are noted in some drug classifications in relation to the reporting of side effects. As an example, women are more prone to develop hypokalemia when taking a diuretic than men. For example, angiotensin-converting enzyme inhibitor and angiotensin receptor blocker should be avoided in women who are or are planning to become pregnant because of the risk to fetal development.

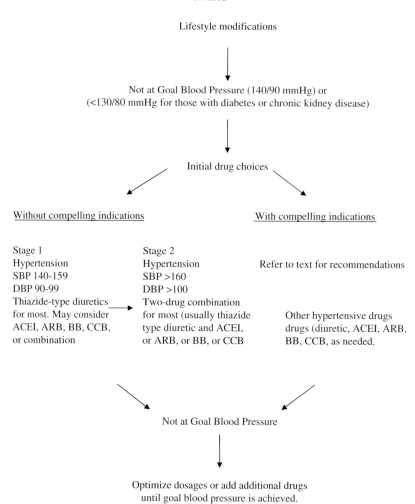

Fig. 1. Algorithm for treatment of hypertension. ACEI, angiotensin-converting enzyme inhibitor; ARB, angiotensin receptor blocker; BB, β-blocker; CCB, calcium channel blocker. (*Adapted from* U.S. Department of Health and Human Services; National Institutes of Health; National Heart, Lung, and Blood Institute. The Seventh Report of the Joint National Committee on Prevention, Detection, Evaluation, and Treatment of High Blood Pressure (JNC 7). Available at: http://www.nhlbi.nih.gov/guidelines/hypertension/. Accessed April 15, 2008; with permission.)

Furthermore, the cough associated with an angiotensin-converting enzyme inhibitor is twice as common in women, and women are more prone to report peripheral edema and hirsutism when placed on a calcium channel blocker. Diuretics are beneficial in the older individual due to the decreased risk of hip fracture [1].

Hypertension in menopausal women

The effect of menopause on blood pressure is not entirely clear. Research shows that women in early adulthood have lower SBP than men, but that as age approaches the sixth decade, the opposite is seen. Supporting evidence shows that menopause may contribute to the rise in blood pressure as women age, possibly related to estrogen withdrawal, overproduction of hormones, weight gain, unknown neurohumoral influences, or a combination of these factors.

The Women's Health Initiative study [6] has followed women taking hormone replacement therapy for several years. This study identified an average 1 mm Hg increase in SBP over 5.6 years among postmenopausal women using

Box 1. Drugs to treat hypertension

Thiazide diuretics
  Inhibit sodium chloride reabsorption in the distal convoluted, decreasing extracellular fluid

Loop diuretics
  Inhibit sodium chloride reabsorption at the loop of Henle, more potent than thiazide diuretics but duration of action is short, and they therefore have less impact on hypertension

Potassium-sparing diuretics
  Reduce potassium and sodium exchange in the distal and collecting tubules

Aldosterone receptor blockers
  Inhibit sodium retaining and potassium excreting activity

β-blockers
  Reduce blood pressure through antagonizing β-adrenergic effect

β-blocker with intrinsic sympathomimetic activity
  Reduce blood pressure through antagonizing β-adrenergic effect

Combined α- and β-blockers
  $\alpha 1$, $\beta 1$, and $\beta 2$ blocking properties result in peripheral vascular dilation and decreased heart rate

Angiotensin-converting enzyme inhibitors
  Inhibit angiotensin-converting enzyme

Angiotensin II antagonists
  Block action of angiotensin

Calcium channel blockers: nondihydropyridines and dihydropyridines
  Block movement of calcium into cells, causing peripheral vasodilation and decreased systemic vascular resistance

α1 blockers
  Block α_1 effect, resulting in peripheral vasodilatation

Central α2 agonists and other centrally acting drugs
  Reduce sympathetic outflow to central nervous system

Direct vasodilators
  Direct arterial vasodilatation, reducing systemic vascular resistance and blood pressure

Box 2. Recommended drug classes for hypertension based on compelling indications

Heart failure
  Diuretics
  β-blockers
  Angiotensin-converting enzyme inhibitors
  Angiotensin receptor blockers
  Aldosterone antagonists

Postmyocardial infarction
  β-blockers
  Angiotensin-converting enzyme inhibitors
  Aldosterone antagonists

High coronary disease risk
  Diuretics
  β-blockers
  Angiotensin-converting enzyme inhibitors
  Calcium channel blockers

Diabetes
  Diuretics
  β-blockers
  Angiotensin-converting enzyme inhibitors
  Angiotensin receptor blockers
  Calcium channel blockers

Chronic kidney disease
  Angiotensin-converting enzyme inhibitors
  Angiotensin receptor blockers

Recurrent stroke prevention
  Diuretics
  Angiotensin-converting enzyme inhibitors

conjugated equine estrogen and medroxyprogesterone acetate compared with the control group. Therefore, the study concluded that hormone replacement therapy has a minimal effect on blood pressure and that therapy should not be withheld in women who have hypertension.

Treating high blood pressure in pregnant or nursing mothers

Before pregnancy, women of childbearing age should have their blood pressure evaluated. Hypertension plays a major role in morbidity and

---

Box 3. Key points relating to hypertension in women

- Age plays a key role in the development of hypertension.
- After 50 years of age, women have a higher incidence of developing hypertension.
- Lifestyle modifications provide the basis for treatment plan.
- Most hypertensive patients will require two or more antihypertensive drugs to reach their goal blood pressure.
- All health care providers have a responsibility to educate and reinforce hypertension management.
- Involvement of the patient and family has a strong correlation to successful management.

---

have a significant effect on the health, financial, and social aspects of individuals. Box 3 lists the key points relating to hypertension in women. Health care providers must involve the patient in each aspect of treatment. Knowledge of the preventive lifestyle modifications and understanding of the medication regime will enable patients to be an active partner in their health needs. Health care providers must listen and respond to concerns and needs of patients and their families. Compliance with the treatment plan remains the key in caring for patients who have hypertension.

mortality of the mother and fetus if not treated. JNC 7 outlines five categories of hypertension in pregnancy:

- Chronic hypertension
- Preeclampsia
- Chronic hypertension with superimposed preeclampsia
- Gestational hypertension
- Transient hypertension

Lifestyle modifications may be the first treatment option. Restrictions on aerobic exercise and weight reduction may be imposed for the health of the mother and fetus. Antihypertensive agents may be selected according to the safety of the fetus. Methyldopa is considered first-line therapy.

Summary

Hypertension remains a major health concern. Preventing and controlling hypertension can

References

[1] U.S. Department of Health and Human Services, National Institutes of Health, National Heart, Lung, and Blood Institute. The Seventh Report of the Joint National Committee on Prevention, Detection, Evaluation, and Treatment of High Blood Pressure. Washington, DC; 2004.

[2] Office of Disease Prevention and Health Promotion, U.S. Department of Health and Human Services. Healthy people 2010. Available at: http//www.healthypeople.gov/. Accessed November 12, 2007.

[3] American Heart Association. Go red for women. Available at: http://goredforwomen.org. Accessed November 12, 2007.

[4] U.S. Department of Health and Human Services, National Institutes of Health, National Heart, Lung, and Blood Institute. Facts about the DASH eating plan. Available at: http://www.nhlbi.nih.gov/health/public/heart/hbp/dash/index.htm. Accessed November 12, 2007.

[5] Adams MP, Josephson DL, Holland LN. Pharmacology for nurses: a pathophysiologic approach. 1st edition. Upper Saddle River (NJ): Pearson Education, Inc; 2005. p. 264–81.

[6] US Department of Health and Human Services. National Institutes of Health. National Heart, Lung, and Blood Institute. Women's Health Initiative (WHI). Available at: http://www.nhlbi.gov/whi. Accessed November 12, 2007.

ELSEVIER
SAUNDERS

Crit Care Nurs Clin N Am 20 (2008) 311–314

CRITICAL CARE
NURSING CLINICS
OF NORTH AMERICA

Women with Dysrhythmia: A Clinical Challenge

Damon B. Cottrell, MS, RN, CCNS, CCRN, CNS-BC, CEN[a],*, Michelle M. Jones, MSN, RN, ACNP-BC, ANP[b]

[a]Cardiology, Washington Hospital Center, 110 Irving Street, NW, 4NE-4082, Washington, DC 20010, USA
[b]Interventional Radiology, Georgetown University Medical Center,
3800 Reservoir Road, NW, Washington, DC 20007, USA

Heart disease is a current and evolving health care issue for women. In the United States, more than 500,000 women die each year of cardiac disease [1], which is the leading cause of death in women [1]. An awareness of the gender differences as they relate to cardiac disease is critically important in the comprehensive care and treatment of women.

Electrocardiographic differences

The electrical conduction system sometimes can be altered by heart disease and lead to dysrhythmia. Therefore, a careful and thorough approach to patient and family history is essential. Paying close attention to symptoms and risk factors while remaining aware of the incidence and prevalence of dysrhythmia in women can be particularly helpful. In performing a physical examination, a critical review of all systems is crucial to detect physical findings that indicate dysrhythmia in the presence or absence of known cardiac disease.

Subtle differences in cardiac rhythm exist between women and men. There is speculation about the cause of the gender differences within ECG readings. Sex hormones, onset of puberty, menstruation, and menopause could be involved, possibly because of the variance in sex hormones during these events. Other possible causes seem to be related to sex-specific differences in the structure of the heart, to differences in the modulation of ion channels within the electrophysiology structures, and to hormonal differences between genders [2,3]. Men have lower resting heart rates than women [3–5]. In addition to the difference in heart rate, studies also have demonstrated that women have longer QT intervals [3,6–8]. Sex hormones may have a role in this prolongation. In men the QT interval shortens most significantly around the age of 20 years, but it increases with age and nears or equals that in women after age 50 years [2,3].

Puberty, the menstrual cycle, and pregnancy also may involved in changes in the electrophysiology status of women. Puberty often marks the onset of symptoms in females who have congenital prolonged QT syndrome. The menstrual cycle seems to affect symptoms of dysrhythmia, which occur much more markedly in the premenstrual phase. Pregnancy may contribute to the onset of ventricular tachycardia or supraventricular tachycardias [2].

Although dysrhythmia occurs in both women and men, nuances specific to women warrant gender-specific evaluation. Careful evaluation including diligent scrutiny of risk factors is key in clinical evaluation. The differences in presenting symptoms, incidence, and outcomes are crucial points of reference in providing care.

Diagnosis

The diagnosis of dysrhythmia is done through patient history, astute assessment, and diagnostic examinations. Often the diagnostic tools are used in combination, because in women symptoms may

* Corresponding author.

E-mail address: damon.b.cottrell@medstar.net
(D.B. Cottrell).

be absent or vague. Women who have significant risk factors should be evaluated even in the absence of significant symptoms.

The 12-lead ECG is a graphic representation of the heart rhythm. It records the electrical activity and specific waveforms that aid in the diagnosis of dysrhythmia, among other problems. In addition to dysrhythmia, it is used to diagnose acute coronary syndromes, electrolyte disturbances, conduction disturbances, and, in some cases, disease or pathology. The ECG commonly is used as the initial diagnostic tool for dysrhythmia.

Another important tool is the Holter monitor, a device worn by the patient for a period of 24 hours or sometimes more. The Holter monitor records patient rhythm over time in much the same manner as the ECG. Patients are asked to engage in normal activities of daily living while keeping a diary of these activities throughout the time frame and to note in the dairy when symptoms are present. This device is an excellent tool for identifying dysrhythmia that is intermittent, paroxysmal, or that is not evident at time of presentation to the health care provider.

Cardiac stress testing is a diagnostic tool that monitors cardiac electrical activity while the patient is stressed, usually by exercise. When physical exercise is not an option, medications such as adenosine or dobutamine may be used to simulate exercise to evaluate the presence of dysrhythmia or underlying coronary artery disease. As with the ECG and ambulatory monitor, electrodes are placed on the chest wall to monitor heart rhythm. An intravenous line usually is present and is used for the administration of medications, if applicable. The heart rhythm is monitored during stress through exercise or during drug administration.

Sonography is used to complete an echocardiogram. This diagnostic tool provides a two-dimensional view of the heart, allowing evaluation of cardiac output, ejection fraction, valve function, cardiac wall movement, and presence or absence of a fistula. An echocardiogram is performed by applying a transducer to the chest wall or through insertion of a device with a sonographic transducer at the distal portion into the esophagus.

An electrophysiology study is a much more complex procedure in which an electrophysiologist uses a catheter to stimulate the heart electrically. This study is used to diagnose rhythm disturbances and to identify problem areas and pathophysiology and for risk stratification. One or more catheters may be inserted into the heart, into the right atrium or right ventricle and the coronary sinus, allowing the evaluation of electrical activity at differing areas or levels within the heart structure.

A head-upright tilt test is helpful in diagnosing autonomic dysfunction and is used frequently in patients who complain of syncope or near syncope. Test protocols differ somewhat, but in most cases the patient is placed on the table in a horizontal position for a short period of time. The table then is tilted upright between 60° and 80°. The patient then is asked to remain still for an additional period of time. The test may involve the administration of isoproterenol or other drugs to aid in evaluation. The ECG is used to monitor rhythm during the examination, and the patient is evaluated for onset of symptoms or changes in blood pressure and heart rate.

Dysrhythmias

"Supraventricular tachycardia" is an umbrella term for a group of dysrhythmias originating in tissue above the atrioventricular (AV) node and ventricles. These dysrhythmias include inappropriate sinus tachycardia, sinoatrial node re-entrant tachycardia, atrial tachycardia, multifocal atrial tachycardia, AV nodal re-entrant tachycardia, and AV re-entrant tachycardia. Technically speaking, it also includes sinus tachycardia, atrial fibrillation, and atrial flutter, because the term refers to any rhythm not of ventricular origin. When these dysrhythmias occur with sudden onset and cessation, the rhythm may be termed "paroxysmal." Symptoms often include palpitations, chest pain, shortness of breath, dyspnea, lightheadedness, and dizziness.

AV nodal re-entrant tachycardia (AVRNT) probably is the most significant supraventricular tachycardia pertaining to women. It represents two thirds of all supraventricular tachycardias and is demonstrated to affect women at a rate of 2:1 [5,9]. Hormones may play a role in AVRNT, particularly during the menstrual cycle [5]. A re-entry circuit within or near the AV node often is the cause. When this phenomenon occurs, symptoms can be present and may include syncope or near syncope. Acute management of this dysrhythmia may include stimulation of vagal response through carotid sinus massage or the Valsalva maneuver. Drugs such as adenosine, beta-blockers, or calcium-channel blockers also may be indicated to control the rate of dysrhythmia and ultimately the symptoms. Catheter ablation is effective in curing the dysrhythmia [8–10].

In both sexes, long QT syndrome may be congenital or acquired [11]. The QT interval has been demonstrated to be longer in families with genotypically characterized long QT syndrome [12], and certain genotypes have been identified with the congenital forms. Risk stratification is helpful in determining the probability of a cardiac event [11]. The acquired form often is associated with medications. A long QT interval corresponds to a prolonged recovery phase or repolarization of the ventricles following contraction. A cardiac cycle initiated early in a patient who has a long QT interval may lead to ventricular dysrhythmias, syncope, and sudden cardiac death.

The risk is ventricular dysrhythmia that can be provoked during the long QT interval. Ventricular tachycardia or torsades de pointes can occur. "Torsades de pointes" is a French term for "twisting of points," named for its polymorphic tachycardia in a short-long-short sequence [11]. This rhythm rarely supports perfusion and may present in syncope, seizure, and cardiac arrest [11].

Treatment of long QT syndrome is focused on prevention and on termination of resulting dysrhythmia when it occurs. Beta-blockers are used for prevention, but certain genotypes are prone to recurrence, and implantable cardiac defibrillators should be considered for these patients [13]. Medications known to prolong the QT interval should be avoided. Pacing also may be indicated as an adjunct to beta-blockers because of the bradycardia or occurrence of pauses seen in patients who have long QT syndrome. When pacing is considered, an implantable cardiac defibrillator often is offered electively [14].

Sudden cardiac death is responsible for up to 400,000 deaths per year in the United States [15]. Overall, up to 80% of victims have a history of cardiac disease, and most victims are male [15]. Sudden cardiac death also occurs without warning of previous heart disease in women [16] but typically occurs 10 to 20 years later in women than in men [8,17]. The predictive risk factors for women—tobacco use, diabetes, and hypertension [3,16]—are different from those in men. Risk factors in women should be evaluated carefully and based on these findings.

Postural orthostatic tachycardia syndrome is characterized by orthostatic intolerance. The defining characteristics are an increase in heart rate with or without a resulting decrease in blood pressure leading to the intolerance. The decrease in blood pressure often is small, or there may be no decrease, leading to an unclear rationale for the symptoms. It is hypothesized that this syndrome is a neurologic disorder. Symptoms are weakness, dizziness, lightheadedness, nausea, headache, tunnel vision, cognitive changes, chest or abdominal pain, sweating, palpitations, and syncope or near syncope [18]. The cause or, more likely, causes are still somewhat unclear. This syndrome can be debilitating and is more common in women [18]. Inappropriate sinus tachycardia (ie, tachycardia without reasonable cause) produces similar symptoms and can be considered an overlapping syndrome [18]. The treatment of postural orthostatic tachycardia syndrome is symptom dependent. In general, patients are encouraged to increase fluid intake to avert hypovolemia. Exercise, reducing the carbohydrate content of meals, and avoiding alcohol also are encouraged. Elastic stockings may increase venous return. If symptoms are severe, drugs such as beta-blockers, fludrocortisone, midodrine, or clonidine may be prescribed. In severe cases, a pacemaker may be considered.

Atrial fibrillation is a common, sustained dysrhythmia in which the ventricular rate is markedly irregular. The incidence of atrial fibrillation increases with age [19]. The atria fibrillate, causing failure of atrial contraction and placing the patient at great risk of thromboembolism and stroke [19]. Symptoms vary greatly. Some patients have no symptoms; others are profoundly affected from a hemodynamic standpoint. Reported symptoms include palpitations, angina, shortness of breath, edema, and activity intolerance. Although atrial fibrillation is more common in men, mortality is higher in women [20]. Because the risk of mortality is more profound in women, aggressive treatment is warranted [8]. Treatment strategies for atrial fibrillation include electrical cardioversion, cardiac ablation, and anticoagulation.

Summary

There are identified differences in the electrophysiologic structure and measurements in women and men. An understanding of these differences and of the increased incidence and prevalence of dysrhythmias in women, the differences in presentation, and the differences in risk factors for these dysrhythmias can help guide treatment decisions. As new knowledge is gained through research, practitioners can provide gender-specific care to women who have or are at increased risk of cardiac dysrhythmia.

References

[1] Mosca L, Appel L, Benjamin E, et al. Evidence-based guidelines for cardiovascular disease prevention in women. Circulation 2004;109:672–93.

[2] Beauregard L-A. Incidence and management of arrhythmias in women. J Gend Specif Med 2002;5: 38–48.

[3] Villareal R, Woodruff A, Massumi A. Gender and cardiac arrhythmias. Tex Heart Inst J 2001;28:265–75.

[4] Liu K, Ballew C, Jacobs D, et al. Ethnic differences in blood pressure, pulse rate, and related characteristics in young adults. The CARDIA study. Hypertension 1989;14:218–26.

[5] Peters RW, Gold MR. The influence of gender on arrhythmias. Cardiol Rev 2004;12:97–105.

[6] Merri M, Bendhorin J, Alberti M, et al. Electrocardiographic quantitation of ventricular repolarization. Circulation 1989;80:1301–8.

[7] Stramba-Badiale M, Locati E, Martinelli A, et al. Gender and the relationship between ventricular repolarization and the cardiac cycle length during 24-h Holter recordings. Eur Heart J 1997;18:1000–6.

[8] Wolbrette D, Patel H. Arrhythmias and women. Curr Opin Cardiol 1999;14:36.

[9] Jayam S, Calkins H. Supraventricular tachycardia. In: Fuster V, Alexander R, O'Rourke R, et al, editors. Hurst's the heart. 11th edition. The McGraw-Hill Companies, Inc.; 2004. p. 855–74.

[10] Jackman W, Beckman K, McClelland J, et al. Treatment of supraventricular tachycardia due to atrioventricular nodal reentry by radiofrequency catheter ablation of slow pathway conduction. N Engl J Med 1992;327:313–8.

[11] Chiang C. Congenital and acquired long QT syndrome. Cardiol Rev 2004;12:222–34.

[12] Lehmann M, Timothy K, Frankovich D, et al. Age-gender influence on the rate-corrected QT interval and the QT-heart rate relation in families with genotypically characterized long QT syndrome. J Am Coll Cardiol 1997;29:93–9.

[13] Priori S, Napolitano C, Schwartz P, et al. Association of long QT syndrome loci and cardiac events among patients treated with beta blockers. JAMA 2004;292:1341–4.

[14] Rho R, Page R. Ventricular arrhythmias. In: Fuster V, Alexander R, O'Rourke R, et al, editors. Hurst's: the heart. 11th edition. York, PA: The McGraw-Hill Companies, Inc.; 2004. p. 875–92.

[15] Rubart M, Zipes D. Mechanisms of sudden cardiac death. J Clin Invest 2005;115:2305–15.

[16] Albert C, Chae C, Grodstein F, et al. Prospective study of sudden cardiac death among women in the united states. Circulation 2003; 107:2096–101.

[17] Kannel W, Wilson P, Offord K, et al. A prospective examination of the Framingham cohort, looking at the incidence and risk factors for SCD in women compared with men. Am Heart J 1998;136:205–12.

[18] Brady P, Low P, Shen W. Inappropriate sinus tachycardia, postural orthostatic tachycardia syndrome, and overlapping syndromes. PACE 2005;28: 1112–21.

[19] Kay G, Plumb V. Atrial fibrillation, atrial flutter, and atrial tachycardia. In: Fuster V, Alexander R, O'Rourke R, et al, editors. Hurst's: the heart. 11th edition. York (PA): The McGraw-Hill Companies, Inc.; 2004. p. 825–54.

[20] Lloyd-Jones D. Beyond the numbers: epidemiology and treatment of atrial fibrillation. Medscape Cardiology 2004. Available at: http://www.medscape.com/viewarticle/494006_print. Accessed December 26, 2007.

ELSEVIER
SAUNDERS

CRITICAL CARE
NURSING CLINICS
OF NORTH AMERICA

Crit Care Nurs Clin N Am 20 (2008) 315–319

Caring for Women Undergoing Cardiac Ablation

Beryl Keegan, RN, MSN/Ed, CCRN, CLNC

*Department of Nursing, Medical Careers Institute, School of Health Science, ECPI College of Technology,
Newport News, VA, USA*

Radiofrequency cardiac ablation (RFCA) has become the treatment of choice for many cardiac arrhythmias that have not responded to medication. RFCA eliminates the arrhythmia by finding an accessible point that either transects and disrupts a reentrant circuit or eliminates a focus. The success rate for RFCA is 90% to 98%. RFCA is used for all tachycardias except for some supraventricular tachycardias. Approximately 15,000 cardiac ablations are performed every year [1,2].

Researchers have found that there is a difference in the prevalence of cardiac arrhythmias between men and women. A woman's heart beats faster than a male's heart; women have a longer QT interval and the incidence of inappropriate sinus tachycardia is a women's arrhythmia. However, women needing treatment for a cardiac arrhythmia tend to wait longer than males; perhaps this is due to waiting until after child bearing years or, that the complaints of palpitations, tachycardia and other arrhythmias are anxiety related. For example, sinus tachycardia, atrioventricular node reentrant tachycardia (AVNRT), inappropriate sinus tachycardia, torsades de pointes, congenital and acquired long QT syndrome, ventricular tachycardia, and sudden cardiac death are common in women. Interestingly atrioventricular reentrant (circus-movement) tachycardia (AVRT), atrial fibrillation (AF), and ventricular fibrillation (VF) happen more often in men [3].

A worldwide survey on cardiac-based AF ablation, coauthored and published earlier this year by Cappato and colleagues [4] summarized the experience from 100 centers with AF catheter ablation programs. The survey found that 52% of the ablations performed were curative, and an additional 24% of patients were able to control the arrhythmias with medication. Cardiac ablation can be used to treat several arrhythmias, with varying success rates. A second ablation procedure was necessary to treat recurring AF in 24.3% of patients, and 3.1% of patients required a third procedure. Complications of cardiac ablation include bleeding, thrombosis, pericardial tamponade, and stroke. Many of these complications are procedure specific, and several complications can be avoided with appropriate nursing care. Quality patient outcomes begin with competent nursing care. Therefore, supportive care and pre- and post-interventional education are vital for patients undergoing the percutaneous cardiac ablation procedure [5].

Description

In the 1990s endeavors at cardiac ablation were modeled after the Maze procedure. In 1998, researchers found that ectopic atrial depolarizations were usually responsible for the initiation of AF and other arrhythmias arose from the pulmonary veins (PV). Another key observation that was made was that ectopic beats responsible for the initiation, and perhaps the maintenance of AF were not randomly located within the heart [6].

Since 2001, significant developments in the field of cardiac electrophysiology have emerged, suggesting that catheter ablation for AF might be successful. The newest approach to cardiac ablation, however, is to advance catheters into the PV via the transeptal approach.

Cardiac ablation is done by inserting catheters through a site in the groin or neck, and with the assistance of fluoroscopy, the electrophysiologist threads 4 electrode catheters through the sheath into the heart via the pulmonary veins. A standard

E-mail address: bphelpskeegan@cox.net

ccnursing.theclinics.com

bipolar or quadripolar catheter will be placed in the right ventricular apex, a quadripolar catheter will go in the coronary sinus, and the ablation catheter, which is floated into the left atrium. Additionally, a pigtail catheter is positioned above the aortic valve that acts as a landmark and removed once arterial access is present to allow for continuous arterial pressure monitoring. Once the damaged site is confirmed, energy is used to destroy a small amount of tissue ending the disturbance of electrical flow through the heart and restoring a healthy heart rhythm [7]. When the catheters arrive at the heart, an electrode on the catheter collects information and electrical measurements are made. Areas observed at this time will be the right atrium, the bundle of His, apex of the right ventricle, and the coronary sinus. This is called "cardiac mapping" and is done to locate the source of the arrhythmia [7].

Atrial fibrillation

More than 2 million people are diagnosed with AF. AF is a chronic disorder which is likely to occur in female patients older than 55 years of age, with hypertension, atrial enlargement, with a previous rheumatic heart disease. AF is distinguished by the absence of coordinated atrial systole. Treatment modalities may include electrical or pharmacologic cardioversion sinus rhythm. However, when these treatment attempts do not work, RFCA has been found to be quite successful, especially in people with paroxysmal AF [8]. RFCA for AF is done by first identifying the foci triggers within the four pulmonary veins (PV). The PVs have been identified as supplying the premature depolarizations that trigger re-entry and rotor waves in the left atrial substrate that may use the PVs as anchor points. And finally, autonomic innervation may also may play a role in AF. The ultimate goal of PV isolation is to create lesions around the perimeter of the PV ostia and interrupt conduction along the sleeves of the atrial tissue that extends from the left atrium into each PV [9]. RFCA has been found to be a relatively safe and successful method in which to treat AF that is refractory to medications and cardioversion.

Atrial flutter

Atrial flutter occurs as the result of a macro-reentrant circuit controlled in the right atrium between two natural endocardial barriers. Additionally, atrial flutter may be the result of an area situated septal to the crista terminalis. Patients may have a chronic or paroxysmal atrial flutter. RFCA is considered an alternative for patients who have atrial flutter that has not responded to pharmacologic therapy. Often a second ablation may be necessary to eradicate the atrial flutter completely. Atrial flutter can be identified on the basis of re-entry around established anatomic landmarks from the tricuspid valve to the inferior vena cava. The success rate is about 92% to 95%, but most patients require repeated procedures [10].

Inappropriate sinus tachycardia

Inappropriate sinus tachycardia is seen in young adult (less than age 40) women, usually in the healthcare profession. While the cause of this rare diagnosis is unknown, inappropriate sinus tachycardia is diagnosed in people having an elevated resting heart rate along with a magnified reaction to stress or exercise. In patients suffering from inappropriate sinus tachycardia, RFCA can be an effective treatment. RFCA for inappropriate sinus tachycardia is done by ablating the sinus node at the area of the earliest activation of the epicardial causing the initial increases in the heart rate. This area is located by the use of mapping with large electrode tip catheters followed by ablating the area of the heart located near the terminal crest. Unfortunately, RFCA for inappropriate sinus tachycardia is usually not successful and may need repeated radiofrequency ablations. Failed cardiac ablations are usually due to a subepicardial location, which is superficial to thick portions of atria musculature in the junction of the superior caval vein with the right atrial appendage [11].

Idiopathic ventricular fibrillation

The source of idiopathic ventricular fibrillation (IVF) is unknown. However, when mapping of the heart is done, the triggers of idiopathic ventricular fibrillation are found in the right and left Purkinijie system. Therefore, the thought of researchers is that IVF is started by a monomorphic early-coupled premature ventricular contraction preceded by a high potential similar to what is seen in the Purkinjie tissue. The potential could represent focal spontaneous activation of local

Purkinjie-like tissue that exhibits concealed firing and at other times results in ventricular activation. RFCA can eradicate these triggers, especially if the heart is normal [12].

Ventricular tachycardia

The treatment of choice for ventricular tachycardia is an implantable cardiac defibrillator and anti-arrhythmic medications. When these measures fail, RFCA may be attempted. When the development of scarring of the myocardium islands of viable muscle cells capable that initiate waves of depolarization occurs due to a myocardial infarction (MI) cause electrical impulses to travel in a circular pattern, causing repeated contractions of the myocardium (called "reentry tachycardia"); there has been some success with ablating of scarred or aneurysmal myocardium. Patients diagnosed as having cardiomyopathy and His-Punkinje system disease may have sustained monomorphic ventricular tachycardia that can be caused by a macro-reentrant circuit that uses the bundle branches. These patients usually complain of shortness of breath or syncopal episodes. Sudden death can result. The most common circuit passes through the right bundle branch and up the left bundle branch. The rates of long-term success are high, but patients may develop heart block.

Patients who have idiopathic ventricular tachycardia or focal tachycardias are good candidates for cardiac ablation. Most idiopathic tachycardias are either outflow tract tachycardias or left idiopathic tachycardias. They usually originate in the right outflow tract. Typically, they are not life threatening, although they can cause syncope. Ablation of these tachycardias is quite successful (about 70%–90%) [13].

Tachycardias

RFCA is used to treat AV nodal reentrant tachycardia, Wolff-Parkinson-White syndrome, and automatic atrial tachycardias. However, complete heart block can be a complication of RFCA for tachycardias. The success rate of RFCA for AV nodal reentrant tachycardia is about 90% to 95% with a complication rate of about 1% [14].

The procedure involves placing the catheters across the tricuspid valve to observe the AV node and in the coronary sinus to map the inferior portion of the right atrium and the left side of the heart. Once in place, the catheter is maneuvered around the mitral valve annulus until the location of the accessory pathway is found. Several attempts may be needed to ablate completely the location of the conduction site [14].

Complications

As with any procedure, RFCA is associated with a set of particular complications. Rates and frequency of complication vary with where the ablation is done. One of the most common complications is a hematoma at the site of access in the thigh. That complication can extend hospital stay, cause pain and discomfort, possibly require a transfusion, and may require surgical repair of a vessel but does not cause long-term disability or problems. The development of a hematoma at the groin site requires immediate direct pressure. To avoid the chance of a hematoma, bed rest must be maintained for at least 4 hours with the head of the bed elevated no more than 30°.

The formation of a pseudoaneurysm is also possible. Any time arterial access is needed for endovascular procedures, cardiac catheterization, or interventional radiology procedures there is an increased rate of femoral pseudoaneurysms, arteriovenous fistulas, and hematomas. The incidence of femoral pseudoaneurysms after an RFAC procedure is about 6%. Typically the pseudoaneurysms thrombose spontaneously after about 4 weeks. If the patient is taking anticoagulants, however, or if the aneurysm is larger than 1.8 cm, it is unlikely to resolve on its own. Repair is done either surgically or with direct thrombin injections [15].

Whenever multiple catheters are used for a cardiac ablation, an arteriovenous fistula may occur. An arteriovenous fistula forms when blood flows directly from an artery into a vein, bypassing the capillaries. If a large acquired arteriovenous fistula is not treated, a sizeable quantity of blood flows from the artery into the venous network. Unfortunately, the vein walls are not sturdy enough to withstand the high pressure, and they extend and swell. The blood flows into the enlarged veins more liberally than if it continued its normal course through the arteries. The blood pressure therefore falls, causing the heart to pump more forcefully and more rapidly, which increases the output of blood and may strain the heart, causing heart failure. Surgery is required to repair an arteriovenous fistula as soon as possible after diagnosis [15].

Postprocedure infections can occur at the sites of a urinary catheter insertion or intubation. Prevention of infection is imperative and can be achieved by hand washing, encouraging the patient to cough and breathe deeply, and timely catheter removal.

A serious complication, which can cause death if left untreated, is cardiac tamponade. Fortunately, the incidence of cardiac tamponade with cardiac ablation is low (about 1%). Cardiac tamponade is caused by excessive fluid within the pericardium that puts weight and pressure on the heart . This pressure does not allow the heart to expand properly; therefore the heart does not fill with normal amounts of blood [16].

The incidence of cardiac tamponade resulting from RFCA is about 1%. The delivery of high energy during RFCA increases the risk of cardiac tamponade. Additionally, the temperature of the catheter tip increases the risk of cardiac tamponade. Cardiac mapping before RFCA may provide the electrophysiologist with enhanced visualization and decrease the incidence of cardiac tamponade [16].

A major complication of RFCA is the possibility of a stroke or transient ischemic attack. The impairment of peripheral blood flow can signify peripheral embolization leading to potential clot formation. This condition can result from lengthy procedure time or bed rest following the procedure. Central embolization can lead to transient ischemic attack or stroke. The risk of stroke can be minimized by the use of systemic heparin. The preprocedure transesophageal echocardiogram will identify any clots present. Any change in neurologic status following the procedure requires an immediate CT scan [17].

Phrenic nerve injury following a cardiac ablation is a well-recognized complication. The right phrenic nerve descends toward the diaphragm and runs anterior to the right PVs. Therefore, phrenic nerve injury occurs most frequently in patients undergoing cardiac ablation for inappropriate sinus tachycardia and AF. Phrenic nerve injury occurs in 2.4% to 24% of patients undergoing a cardiac ablation; most patients attain at least partial recovery in 3 months. The most common symptoms of phrenic nerve injury are shortness of breath, cough, hiccups, pneumonia, or pleural effusion.

Radiofrequency energy delivered around the PVs can cause severe stenosis, which often progresses to partial loss of flow or total obstruction of one or several vessels. The clinical symptoms of PV stenosis are quite variable, including chest pain, dyspnea, cough, hemoptysis, recurrent lung infection, and pulmonary hypertension [18]. The anatomy of the PVs can vary significantly from patient to patient. A preprocedure spiral CT of the chest allows visualization of the PVs, which play such an important role in triggering AF.

Rupture of the superior vena cava is an infrequent but life-threatening complication that usually is caused by frequent or repeated procedures. Percutaneous balloon dilation can be attempted and is successful in some cases, but immediate open-heart surgery is required if dilation is not successful [19].

Other possible complications include accidental perforation of the coronary sinus or chamber, a hemopericardium, or trauma. Collateral damage that can occur includes complete heart blockage, myocardial infarction, heart failure, pleural effusion, or cardiogenic shock.

Nursing care

Before the procedure the cardiologist may order a CT scan to identify the location of the PVs and other structures within the chest. The use of antiarrhythmic, anticoagulation, and antiplatelet medications is stopped several days before the procedure. A transesophageal echocardiogram is obtained to rule out an atrial thrombus. Any abnormal blood chemistries must be corrected before the procedure to reduce the risk of ventricular irritability. Additionally, any elevation in the serum urea nitrogen or creatine level may suggest pre-existing renal insufficiency and may predispose the patient to developing renal ischemia secondary to the use of contrast dye [17].

Nursing care is extremely important and involves frequent monitoring of vital signs and groin sites. Vital signs and oxygen saturation are monitored every 15 minutes during the first hour and then every 2 hours for 12 hours. The patient should not be allowed to flex the affected hip for 3 to 5 hours. If the artery is used, the leg must be kept straight for 6 hours, and the patient must lie flat for 4 to 6 hours. The doctor will remove the catheters and apply pressure to the insertion sites, but sites in the groin must be monitored for any signs of bleeding. If bleeding does occur, the immediate application of direct pressure is vital. Any decrease in blood pressure must be treated with fluids. If the blood pressure does not respond to fluid administration, an ECG should be done to assess for a pleural effusion. On discharge the patient is instructed about activity, medications, and follow-up [17].

Summary

Historically, health care professionals have not provided women with treatment equal that given men. Only recently has any research investigated the gender differences in health care. Although the arrhythmias treated by RFCA may be differ in men and women, pre- and postprocedure nursing care for the patient undergoing RFCA does not. No research indicates that either gender has more complications than the other. Caring for patients as individuals and being knowledgeable about the possible complications associated with RFCA are imperative in providing successful outcomes.

References

[1] Magnana AR, Woolett I, Garan H. Catheter ablation for the treatment of atrial fibrillation. J Card Surg 2004;19(3):188–95.

[2] Chapnick MT, Bauer J. Technology today radiofrequency cardiac ablation. RN 2005;68(10):40–5.

[3] Villareal RP, Woodruff AL, Massumi A. Gender and cardiac arrhythmias. Tex Heart Inst J 2001; 28(4):265–75.

[4] Cappato R, Calkins H, Chen SA, et al. Worldwide survey on the methods, efficacy, and safety of catheter ablation for human atrial fibrillation. Circulation 2005;111(9):1100–5.

[5] Thompson EJ, Reich DA, Meadow JL. Radiofrequency ablation in the pulmonary veins for paroxysmal drug-resistant atrial fibrillation. Dimens Crit Care Nurs 2004;23(6):255–63.

[6] Agarwal A, York M, Kantharia BK, et al. Atrial fibrillation: modern concepts and management. Annl Rev Med 2005;56(1):475–94.

[7] Thompson EJ, Reich DA, Meadow L. Radiofrequency ablation in the pulmonary veins for paroxysmal drug-resistant atrial fibrillation. Dimens Crit Care Nurs 2004;23(6):9:255–63.

[8] Bentz B. Gaining control over A-fib. RN 2006; 69(12):35–8.

[9] Pappone C, Santinelli V. The who, what, why, and how-to guide for circumferential pulmonary vein ablation. J Cardiovasc Electrophysiol 2004;15(10): 1226–30.

[10] DaCosta A, Mourot S, Romeyer-Bouchard C, et al. Anatomic and electrophysiological differences between chronic and paroxysmal forms of common atrial flutter and comparison with controls. Pacing Clin Electrophysiol 2004;27:1202–11.

[11] Koplan BA, Parkash R, Couper G. Combined epicardial-endocardial approach to ablation of inappropriate sinus tachycardia. J Cardiovasc Electrophysiol 2004;15:237–40.

[12] Betts TR, Yue A, Roberts PR, et al. Radiofrequency ablation of idiopathic ventricular fibrillation guided by noncontact mapping. J Cardiovasc Electrophysiol 2004;15(8):957–9.

[13] Agarwal A, et al. Atrial fibrillation: modern concepts and management. Annu Rev Med 2005;56(1): 475–95.

[14] Satti SD, Epstein LP. Cardiologic interventional therapy for atrial and ventricular arrhythmias. Cardiac surgery in the adult. New York: McGraw-Hill; 2003.

[15] Kendrick AS, Sprouse LR II. Repair of a combined femoral pseudoaneurysm and arteriovenous fistula using a covered stent graft. Am Surg 2007;73(3): 227–9.

[16] Hsu L, Jais P, Hocini M, et al. Incidence and prevention of cardiac tamponade complicating ablation for atrial fibrillation. Pacing Clin Electrophysiol 2005; 28(1):106–9.

[17] Zak J. Mapping of ventricular tachycardia. Crit Care Nurse 2006;26(5):13–5.

[18] Bai R, Patel D, Blasé L, et al. Phrenic nerve injury. Should we worry about this complication? J Cardiovasc Electrophysiol 2006;17(9):944–8.

[19] Oshima K, Takahashi T, Ishikawa S, et al. Superior vena cava rupture caused during balloon dilation for treatment of SVC syndrome due to repetitive catheter ablation. Angiology 2007;57(2):247–9.

ELSEVIER
SAUNDERS

Crit Care Nurs Clin N Am 20 (2008) 321–326

CRITICAL CARE
NURSING CLINICS
OF NORTH AMERICA

Hypothermic Coma: Catapulting Evidence-Based Research Into Everyday Practice

Lynn Smith Schnautz, RN, MSN, CCRN, CCNS, NP-C[a,b,]*,
Dawn Rowley, RN[a]

[a]Deaconess Hospital, Evansville, IN, USA
[b]Integrity Family Physicians, Evansville, IN, USA

Misty's red dress

A 26-year-old white woman is brought to the emergency room by ambulance (Fig. 1). She is unresponsive, intubated, and placed on mechanical ventilation. She is accompanied by her friend, who states that the patient began a jogging exercise program that morning. The patient jogged a block, walked a block, jogged a block, walked a block, and then collapsed.

Her friend called 911 and started cardiopulmonary resuscitation (CPR) immediately. When the emergency medical service arrived, she was found to be in ventricular fibrillation and was defibrillated twice before converting to normal sinus rhythm. Time of witnessed collapse to stabilization in the field was less than 15 minutes, with transport time to the emergency room (ER) less than 30 minutes from collapse to hospitalization. She was stabilized in the ER then transferred to the cardiovascular intensive care unit (ICU).

Initial assessment in the ICU showed a 26-year-old white woman who looked her stated age, was unresponsive, had score of 5T or less on the Glasgow Coma Scale, showed a normal sinus rhythm (NSR) on the monitor, and was placed on mechanical ventilation. According to family, she had a history of cardiac problems, including coronary artery disease, hyperlipidemia, and hypertension. She underwent a coronary angiogram 2.5 years before, which showed significant coronary disease with occlusion of the left mid anterior descending artery, proximal right coronary artery, and distal left main coronary artery. Her cardiologist decided to treat her medically because of her age.

Current medications on admission included atenolol, 25 mg daily, Lipitor, 80 mg daily, isosorbide as needed, and aspirin, 81 mg daily. The patient had recently started walking and engaging in some exercise. She was having some problems with dizziness, especially early in the morning, and her cardiologist advised her not to increase her activity or to begin jogging. The ICU nurses contacted the Indiana Organ Procurement Organization for potential donation referral.

Based on Misty's presentation, the attending physician and nursing staff determined that she was a candidate for hypothermic coma, an experimental procedure that had been well documented in the research literature. This institution had used this procedure successfully once before, and the patient was determined to be an ideal candidate.

This article discusses how a group of critical care nurses, a pulmonologist, and a pharmacist developed a hypothermic coma protocol for treating patients after cardiac arrest, and discusses the conceptual model used for translating evidence into clinical practice.

Conceptual model for translating evidence into clinical practice

Rosswurm and Larrabee proposed a model for guiding nurses through a systematic process for the change to evidence-based practice. This model

---

* Corresponding author.
E-mail address: lynn_schnautz@deaconess.com
(L.S. Schnautz).

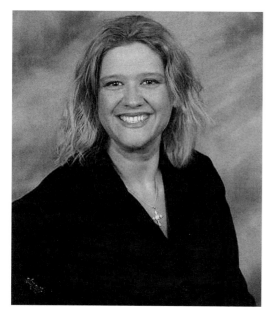

Fig. 1. A patient at Deaconess Hospital (Misty Baldwin) who was placed in a hypothermic coma after cardiac arrest.

recognized that translating research into practice requires a solid grounding in change theory, principles of research use, and use of standardized nomenclature. The model has six phases [1]:

1. Assess the need for change in practice
2. Link the problem with interventions and outcomes
3. Synthesize the best evidence
4. Design a change in practice
5. Implement and evaluate the practice
6. Integrate and maintain the practice change

Assess the need for change in practice

Cardiac arrest outside the hospital is a major cause of unexpected death in developed countries, with survival rates ranging from less than 5% to 35%. In patients who are initially resuscitated, anoxic neurologic injury is an important cause of morbidity and mortality.

Currently, treatment of patients in a coma after resuscitation from out-of-hospital cardiac arrest is largely supportive. Because cerebral ischemia may persist for some hours after resuscitation, the use of induced hypothermia to decrease cerebral oxygen demand has been proposed as a treatment option [2].

Assessing the need for change in practice, Misty could have been treated supportively and

may have been an ideal candidate for organ procurement, or would have experienced permanent anoxic injury. Exploring evidence-based research and implementing hypothermia may allow for better neurologic outcomes.

Link the problem with interventions and outcomes

Currently, patients who have undergone cardiac arrest who are comatose on admission present a challenge. According to the literature, treatment with induced hypothermia has better neurologic outcomes than supportive treatment.

Synthesize the best evidence

History of hypothermia

The first documented medical use of hypothermia was in 1937, when Dr. Faye Temple cooled a female patient to 32°C (89.6°F) to relieve the symptoms of metastatic cancer. Dr. Temple proposed that by cooling a patient's core body temperature to 32°C, cells would not divide, thereby halting the production of cancer. Dr. Temple placed her patients in a barbiturate coma before she packed them on ice for 24 hours, then passively rewarmed them. She performed the procedure on 123 patients who had cancer but concluded that using induced hypothermia had no apparent effect on cancer progression [3].

In 1941, Smith and Faye observed that induced hypothermia improved the conscious state of a patient who had head injury. In the 1950s, Bigelow and colleagues introduced moderate hypothermia, 28°C (82.4°F) to 32°C (89.6°F), to protect the brain from ischemia during cardiac surgical procedures; this remains the current practice. From the 1960s to 1990s, few clinical studies were published on the clinical use of induced hypothermia [3].

Normothermia, the body's normal temperature, ranges between 37°C (98.6°F) and 38°C (100.4°F). In the context of induced hypothermia, this range is often used as the end point for rewarming. Mild hypothermia is defined as a body temperature between 33°C (91.4°F) and 36°C (98.6°F). Several clinical studies on induced hypothermia after cardiac arrest or traumatic brain injury had 32°C (89.6°F) to 34°C (93.2°F), considered mild-to-moderate hypothermia, as the goal of treatment [4].

When a patient is resuscitated, reperfusion initiates a series of chemical reactions that can continue for up to 24 hours, possibly causing significant inflammation in the brain. Inducing mild hypothermia decreases intracranial pressure, the cerebral metabolic rate, and the brain's demand for oxygen consumption. In addition, it is believed to suppress many chemical reactions associated with reperfusion injury, including free radical production, excitatory amino acid release, and calcium shifts, which can then lead to mitochondrial damage and apoptosis. The end result is that patients have a better chance of recovering with their neurologic function intact [5,6].

Research

Two landmark randomized, controlled studies—one in Europe and one in Australia—were published in the February 2002 issue of the *New England Journal of Medicine*. In the European study, participants were included if they experienced a witnessed, out-of-hospital cardiac arrest, with ventricular fibrillation (or nonperfusing ventricular tachycardia) as the presenting rhythm, with successful CPR in less than 60 minutes, and an interval between cardiac arrest and the initiation of cardiopulmonary resuscitation of 5 to 15 minutes [7]. Patients who had any of the following were excluded from the study:

"A tympanic-membrane temperature below 30°C on admission, a comatose state before the cardiac arrest due to the administration of drugs that depress the central nervous system, pregnancy, response to verbal commands after the return of spontaneous circulation and before randomization, evidence of hypotension (mean arterial pressure, less than 60 mm Hg) for more than 30 minutes after the return of spontaneous circulation and before randomization, evidence of hypoxemia (arterial oxygen saturation, less than 85 percent) for more than 15 minutes after the return of spontaneous circulation and before randomization, a terminal illness that preceded the arrest, factors that made participation in follow-up unlikely, enrollment in another study, the occurrence of cardiac arrest after the arrival of emergency medical personnel, or a known preexisting coagulopathy [7]."

At arrest, patients were randomized into either hypothermia or normothermia groups (N = 275). Both groups underwent standard intensive care. In the hypothermia group, cooling was induced with a cooling blanket as soon as possible to a goal temperature of between 32°C (89.4°F) and 34°C (93.2°F) within 4 hours, determined through bladder temperature. Ice packs were used in patients not meeting the goal temperature. Patients were mechanically ventilated and sedated with midazolam, fentanyl, and pancuronium.

Hypothermia was maintained for 24 hours, followed by passive rewarming.

The primary end point was a favorable neurologic outcome within 6 months (defined as "good recovery" or "moderate disability" on a five-point scale), meaning that the patient had the ability to live independently and work part-time. Secondary end points included mortality at 6 months and the frequency of complications, such as pneumonia, sepsis, or pressure ulcers, in the first several days after the event [7].

Favorable neurologic outcomes after 6 months were seen in 55% of the patients in the hypothermia group, compared with 39% in the normothermic group. In addition, the mortality rate in the hypothermia group was lower than that in the normothermia group (41% versus 55%) [7].

The Australian study produced comparable results, although the researchers used slightly different inclusion criteria, methods, and a smaller subject sample (N = 77). The goal temperature was reached in 2 hours and the patients were maintained in the hypothermic coma at 33°C (91.4°F) for only 12 hours. The rate of favorable outcomes (defined as discharge home or to rehabilitation) was 49% in the hypothermic group verses 26% in the normothermic group. Death rates were 51% in the hypothermic group and 68% in the normothermic group [2].

Contraindications

The two clinical studies discussed earlier concluded that induced hypothermia effectively improves neurologic outcomes in a select group of patients. It is contraindicated in most patients who experienced cardiac arrest. In fact, more than 90% of patients screened for inclusion in the European study did not meet inclusion criteria.

Complications from induced hypothermia were identified in both studies. In the Australian study, patients in the hypothermia group had lower cardiac indices, greater systemic vascular resistance, and more hyperglycemia than those in the normothermia group. Other possible complications include coagulopathy, electrolyte abnormalities, decreased immune function, and altered drug metabolism [8].

Design a change in practice

Protocol

A group consisting of a pulmonologist, a clinical nurse specialist, a pharmacist, and critical care nurses (Fig. 2) at Deaconess Hospital in

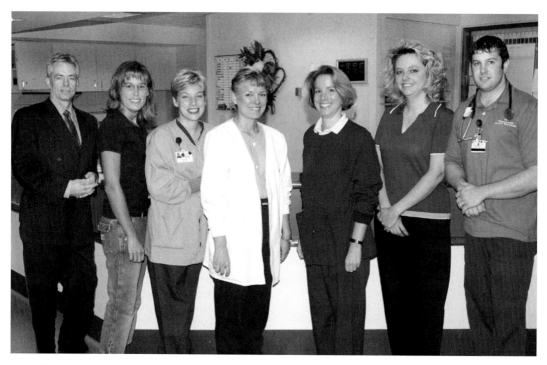

Fig. 2. Hypothermic coma: catapulting evidence-based research into everyday practice. Members of the Deaconess Hospital Hypothermic Coma Team (left to right): Dr. David Harris; Dawn Rowley, RN; Tracy Maglis, RN; Tricia Maas, RN, Lynn Schnautz, RN, MSN, CCRN, CCNS; Meredith Petty, PharmD.; Eric Glines, RN, MSN, ACNP. (*Courtesy of Dave Waller*).

Evansville, Indiana, developed a protocol based on the research of these two landmark studies. The protocol should be initiated within 6 hours of patient admission. The patient must display the following inclusion criteria to be placed in the hypothermic coma:

1. Within 1 hour from onset, one of the following:
   a. Cardiac arrest
   b. Ventricular fibrillation
   c. Nonperfusing ventricular tachycardia

2. Mean arterial pressure of 60 mm Hg or greater with or without the use of vasopressors
3. Persistent coma after return of spontaneous cardiac circulation as evidenced by:
   a. Neurologic examination that shows comatose patient who has a score of 5T or less on Glasgow Coma Scale
   or
   b. Neurologic examination that shows patient unresponsive to verbal stimuli with a score of 5T or less on Glasgow Coma Scale

Patients are excluded from the protocol if any of the following are identified: (1) responsive and following commands, (2) tympanic-membrane temperature less then 30°C on admission, (3) comatose state before cardiac arrest caused by administration of drugs that depress the central nervous system, (4) pregnancy, (5) terminal illness that preceded the arrest, or (6) known preexisting coagulopathy.

When patients meet inclusion criteria for hypothermic coma, ice packs are applied to the neck, groin, and axillae. They are then placed on a cooling blanket (one blanket below and one on top) and cooled to a rectal body temperature of 32°C (89.6°) to 34°C (93.2°F) for 12 to 24 hours. All other goal-directed therapeutic treatment related to admitting diagnosis is initiated (ie, thrombolytics, cardiac catheterization) as indicated.

Patients are maintained on mechanical ventilation, and a pulmonary consultation is obtained. A midazolam infusion is used for short-term sedation during the induced hypothermia. Fentanyl, 50 to 100 µg intravenously, may be given every 15 to 60 minutes as needed for pain management. A modified version of the Rider

Sedation-Agitation Scale is used to help monitor the patient. The patient is paralyzed with cis-atracurium intravenously to prevent shivering because it is less vagolytic than other neuromuscular blocking agents and does not accumulate as readily in the liver and kidneys of patients who have renal or hepatic disease. The cisatracurium drip is titrated according to the neuromuscular blockage train-of-four monitoring [4].

Treatment termination consists of removing ice packs and cooling blankets after 12 to 24 hours of induced hypothermia per physician recommendation. The patient is allowed to rewarm passively by room temperature. When the patient's body temperature is greater than 35.5°C, cisatracurium is discontinued, followed by midazolam then fentanyl. The patient is then weaned from mechanical ventilation.

Implement and evaluate the practice

Education

Initially the Hypothermic Coma Protocol Team presented the research-based protocol to the ER physicians and nurses, then to each of the intensive care nurses. Local emergency medical services were also educated on the protocol and inclusion and exclusion criteria, and early initiation of the protocol was instituted. The protocol was presented to the hospital physicians during monthly grand rounds.

Outcomes

In its first year of use, 10 patients met the criteria for use of the hypothermic coma protocol at Deaconess Hospital, 9 of whom survived and experienced complete neurologic recovery. At this writing, the protocol has been in use for 5 years, with more than 40 patients experiencing complete neurologic recovery.

Evidence from the European and Australian research studies was so compelling that the International Liaison Committee in 2003 recommended using hypothermic coma to treat all patients who experienced out-of-hospital cardiac arrest. The recommendations were also included in the 2005 American Heart Association Advanced Cardiac Life Support Guidelines for treating all patients who experience out-of-hospital cardiac arrest.

Hypothermic coma is also showing promising results with patients who experienced brain and spinal cord injury. When the Buffalo Bill's tight-end, Kevin Everett, was injured while playing football in September 2007, hypothermia was initiated immediately during transport to the hospital. Mr. Everett's initial injuries showed a C3–C4 direct compression injury with paralysis from his shoulders and below. Mr. Everett's body temperature was cooled to 33°C (92°F) to protect his brain and spinal cord. The doctors reported that after hypothermia, Mr. Everett regained some use of his arms and legs [9]. Additional success stories have also been featured nationally in the news.

Integrate and maintain the practice change

The protocol has been updated since its initial inception 5 years ago. The protocol is currently presented during the hospital's yearly Critical Care Classes to all new graduates, and monthly during Critical Care Education Day to all of the critical care nurses. The Hypothermic Coma Protocol team has spoken locally, regionally, and nationally at nursing seminars about the development and research outcomes of the protocol.

The success of the hypothermic coma team has been amazing. The team published a case study in the February 2005 issue of the American Journal of Nursing, and has received the 2006 American Heartsaver Award and the 2006 American Association of Critical Care Nurses Circle of Excellence Datascope Excellence in Collaboration Nurse-Physician Award.

Misty's red dress: conclusion

Misty was placed in the hypothermic coma for 24 hours. It took her 12 hours to obtain a core body temperature of 33°C. She was taken to the cardiac catheterization laboratory were her cardiologist determined that she had triple vessel disease. All other supportive therapy was continued as outlined in the protocol.

She was passively rewarmed after 24 hours, sedation and paralytics were discontinued, and she was extubated from the ventilator. She was completely neurologically intact; however, she had no recollection of the events that transpired while she was hospitalized. She underwent coronary artery bypass grafting of three vessels 1 week later.

Today she is living a heart-healthy life style, working as a print estimator, and is a speaker for the Mended Hearts Program (a support group for patients who undergo open heart surgery) at Deaconess Hospital. Misty's story has also been featured in Redbook.

Summary

The use of hypothermic coma has been well established in the literature for patients who experienced cardiac arrest who exhibit ventricular fibrillation or ventricular tachycardia. Its use is recommended by the American Heart Association immediately on transportation to the hospital for all out-of-hospital ventricular fibrillation. Early recognition and use of hypothermia in patients who experienced cardiac arrest has positive outcomes. Hypothermia shows promising results for future use in patients who experienced brain and spinal cord injury. Nurses using Rosswurm and Larrabee's conceptual model are guided through a systematic approach to translating evidence-based research into everyday clinical practice.

Acknowledgment

The authors would like to thank Dr. David Harris; Eric Glines, RN, MSN, ACNP; and Meredith Petty, PharmD for their hard work and dedication in the development and education of this protocol for the past 5 years. Thank you to the doctors and nurses at Deaconess Hospital for using this evidence-based protocol, which has benefited many patients in the Tri-State Community. Many thanks to Drs. Bernard and Holzer for their pioneering research, which has forever changed the lives for many individuals, families, and communities with this revolutionary treatment of patients who experienced cardiac arrest.

References

[1] Conceptual model for translating evidence into clinical practice 2008. Available at: www.medscape.com/viewarticle/514532_5. Accessed January 30, 2008.

[2] Bernard SA, Gray TW, Buist MD, et al. Treatment of comatose survivors of out-of-hospital cardiac arrest with induced hypothermia. N Engl J Med 2002;346(8):557–63.

[3] Bernard SA, Buist M. Induced hypothermia in critical care medicine: a review. Critical Care Medicine 2003;31(7):2041–51.

[4] Schnautz L, Glines E, Rowley D, et al. To freeze or not to freeze: inducing hypothermic coma after cardiac arrest. Am J Nurs 2005;105(2):72AA–72DD.

[5] Nolan JP, Morley PT, Vanden Hoek TL, et al. Therapeutic hypothermia after cardiac arrest: an advisory statement by the advanced life support task force of the international liaison committee on resuscitation. Circulation 2003;108(1):118.

[6] American Heart Association. American heart association outlines "chilling" plan to prevent brain damage after cardiac arrest. 2003 Available at: www.americanheart.org/presenter.jhtml?idenifier=3013397. Accessed January 30, 2008.

[7] Hypothermia after Cardiac Arrest Study Group. Mild therapeutic hypothermia to improve the neurologic outcome after cardiac arrest. N Engl J Med 2002;346(8):549–56.

[8] Polderman KH. Application of therapeutic hypothermia in the intensive car unit. Opportunities and pitfalls of a promising treatment modality—part 2: practical aspects and side effects. Intensive Care Med 2004;30(5):757–69.

[9] Higgins M. Football: optimism on Kevin Everett, NFL player, spinal cord injury. (September 12, 2007). Available at: http://www.nytimes.com/2007/09/11/sports/football/11everett.html. Accessed December 30, 2007.

ELSEVIER
SAUNDERS

CRITICAL CARE
NURSING CLINICS
OF NORTH AMERICA

Crit Care Nurs Clin N Am 20 (2008) 327–341

Heart Failure: It's Not Just for Men

Angela L. Pruitt, MSN, RN, CNS

Cardiovascular Renal Care Center, Deaconess Hospital, Inc., 600 Mary Street, Evansville, IN 47740, USA

What do we know about women and heart failure?

Statistics

Coronary heart disease is the leading cause of morbidity and mortality in women. One in four women dies of heart disease, whereas 1 in 30 dies of breast cancer. Twenty-three percent of women who experience a myocardial infarction (MI) die within 1 year. Within 6 years of having an MI, 46% of women develop disabling heart failure (HF), compared with 25% of men [1–3].

Women older than 40 years who have not had a previous MI have a one in six lifetime risk of developing HF, compared with risk of one in nine for men. The American Heart Association (AHA) 2004 statistics for cardiovascular disease in women reveal the mortality from heart disease for all ages was 39% in men and 61.1% in women. The prevalence is higher in black women (3.3%) than in white women (2.1%) [4].

Cost of care, length of stay, and readmission rates

HF is a global health issue. As life expectancy increases, so does the incidence and prevalence of HF. Health care providers need to deal with the rising trends of diabetes, hypertension (HTN), and obesity, because these diseases, which are risk factors for HF, place a huge burden on health care expenditures [5].

It is estimated that in 2008 the costs for health care (direct costs) and lost productivity (indirect costs) for all cardiovascular disease and stroke in the United States will be $448.5 billion. Projections for 2008 total hospital costs are $140.1 billion, compared with the 2007 estimated hospital costs of $89 billion for all cancer. The 2008 estimated direct and indirect costs for HF are $34.8 billion [6].

HF has increased in severity and is the leading cause of all hospitalizations for patients older than 65 years. Recurrent HF is the most common cause for readmission of elderly patients, and 50% of patients age 65 years and older who have HF are readmitted within 6 months of discharge [2]. In the period from 1979 to 2005, HF hospital discharges increased by 171%, from 400,000 to 1,084,000 [6].

Definition of heart failure

HF is end-stage cardiac disease and progressive in nature. The cardiovascular system weakens after primary damage occurs from a chronic increase in volume or pressure load or by an increase in metabolic demand on the myocardium, such as found with HTN, an MI, or a viral infection. The cardiovascular system loses the ability to provide an adequate supply of nutrients and oxygenated arterial blood to the organs and tissues and to return venous blood to the lungs through the right heart. As the heart enlarges, the ventricles become stiff, increasing resistance and decreasing contractility, and thus reducing cardiac output. Blood flows more slowly through the kidneys, which in turn compensate for the decreased cardiac output by triggering the retention of sodium and water, thus contributing to the progression of edema.

Reported symptoms vary depending on whether there is left-heart or right-heart involvement. In left-sided HF, cardiac output is decreased systemically, causing a backup of blood into the lungs and resulting in pulmonary edema. As venous blood returns to a failing right heart, the blood cannot be pumped adequately to the pulmonary system. Therefore blood accumulates in the peripheral vascular system, causing venous pooling in the extremities.

E-mail address: angela_pruitt@deaconess.com

Diastolic HF is defined as HF with a normal ejection fraction of 50% or greater, (HFNEF), which has a better prognosis than systolic HF, that is, HF with a reduced ejection fraction of 40% or less (HFREF). HFNEF becomes more prevalent in women as age increases. The annual mortality rate is 8% to 9% for HFNEF and 15% to 19% for HFREF [7]. HF progresses to death. Sudden cardiac death is six to nine times more common in women than in the general population [6].

Viewed as a man's disease

In the past, clinical research included more men than women, but results were generalized to the entire population to formulate recommended guidelines for medical care. In the early 1990s, the inequalities in clinical research studies led to the birth of the Women's Health Initiative. This 15-year project included women and ethnic minorities to look at the leading causes of illness in women: heart disease, breast and colorectal cancer, and osteoporosis in postmenopausal women [8].

Before the Women's Health Initiative, the Framingham Heart Study conducted by the National Heart Lung and Blood Institute was the foremost study focusing on heart disease in the United States. The 44-year follow-up of the Framingham Heart Study indicated that the incidence of HF in persons older than 65 years has risen to 10 per 1000 population. Deaths from HF increased by 28%, although the death rate between 1994 and 2004 declined by 2.0% [2].

Eighty percent of men and 70% of women diagnosed with HF at an age younger than 65 years die within 8 years of diagnosis. Although the survival rate is lower in men, fewer than 15% of women who have HF survive more than 8 to 12 years, and women's 1-year morality rate is 20% [6].

Causes and risk factors for heart failure in women

The common risk factors and causes for development of HF are outlined in Box 1.

To improve early identification of HF in women, physicians, advanced health care practitioners, and nurses need to focus on the rising trend of diabetes, HTN, and obesity. According to Mayo Clinic researchers, the prevalence of diabetes increases 3.8% every year. Diabetic women who have an elevated body mass index (BMI) or reduced creatinine clearance rate are at highest risk. The incidence in diabetic patients who have no other risk factors is 3.0% and

---

Box 1. Risk factors and causes for heart failure

Risk factors
- Age 65 years or older (for women)
- African American race
- Family history of heart failure
- Diabetes
- Smoking
- High blood pressure
- Hypertension
- Irregular heart beat
- Sedentary lifestyle
- Increased BMI or obesity
- Eating foods high in fat and cholesterol
- High cholesterol and low-density lipoprotein levels
- Low high-density lipoprotein levels
- Drug abuse, especially cocaine, methamphetamine
- Heavy consumption or abuse of alcohol

Causes of heart failure
- Coronary artery disease
- Myocardial infarction
- Atrial fibrillation
- Valvular disease
- Viral infection, including HIV
- Dilated cardiomyopathy: enlarged heart
    - Coronary artery disease; myocardial infarction; diabetes; thyroid disease; alcohol, cocaine, amphetamines abuse; chemotherapeutic agents (doxorubicin, daunorubicin)
- Hypertrophic cardiomyopathy: heart muscle thickens, left ventricle enlarges
    - Hypertension; congenital; age related
- Restrictive cardiomyopathy: stiff, ridged ventricles (scar tissue)
    - Hemochromatosis; amyloidosis; sarcoidosis; connective tissue disorders
- Severe lung disease, kidney failure, anemia

increases significantly to 8.2% if three or more risk factors are present [3]. Diabetes is the strongest risk factor, but HTN is more predictive of HF in women [7]. Diabetes is a disease that requires lifestyle modification and treatment with pharmacotherapy. Diligent monitoring and working with a health care provider may help lower a hemoglobin A_{1C} that is higher than 7% [5].

Seventy-five percent of patients who have HF have precursor HTN [4], and the lifetime risk of HF is twice as great for a person who has a blood pressure higher than 160/90 mm Hg than for a person who has a blood pressure of 140/90 mm Hg [9]. The Women's Health Initiative 7.7-year follow-up of postmenopausal women age 50 to 79 years found the baseline rate of prehypertension in this population was 38.8%, and 34.9% of this population had HTN. The progression from a normal blood pressure to hypertension was paralleled by an increased prevalence in diabetes, greater BMI, and hypercholesterolemia. Prehypertension increased the risk of MI, stroke, HF, and cardiovascular death in postmenopausal women, validating the importance of early global risk assessment and aggressive management [10].

Hypertension can be managed by maintaining a healthy BMI, daily exercise, moderation in alcohol consumption, and by changing dietary habits. What happens if these interventions do not work? When blood pressure is higher than 140/90 mm Hg (or > 130/80 mm Hg in patients who have diabetes or chronic kidney disease), a thiazide diuretic is prescribed, unless contraindicated. At-risk women may require beta-blockers, angiotensin-converting enzyme inhibitors, and/or angiotensin-receptor blockers with a thiazide diuretic to achieve goal blood pressure [5].

Women need to be proactive and know their lipid levels, blood pressure, glucose, BMI, and waist circumference (Box 2).

Ethnicity

Ethnicity brings to light associated risk factors attributable to socioeconomic status and geographic location. The Study of Women's Health Across the Nation looked at premenopausal women, 42 to 52 years of age. The educational level was lowest in Hispanic women and highest in white women. Chinese and Japanese women had the lowest BMIs, while African American women had the highest BMIs, continued to smoke, and were being treated with antihypertensives. High-density lipoprotein (HDL) cholesterol levels were

---

> **Box 2. Normal levels for lipids, blood pressure, glucose, body mass index, and waist circumference**
>
> Glucose: Hemoglobin A_{1C} < 7% without significant hypoglycemia
> Blood pressure: < 120/80 mm Hg
> Lipid levels:
>   Low-density lipoprotein cholesterol < 100 mg/dL
>   High-density lipoprotein cholesterol > 50 mg/dL
>   Triglycerides < 150 mg/dL
> Body mass index: Maintain between 18.5 and 24.9
> Waist circumference: ≤ 35 inches

---

highest among Chinese and Japanese women and lowest in African American and Hispanic women; white women sustained an intermediate level. Chinese women had favorable Framingham risk scores, whereas African American and Hispanic women had less favorable scores [11].

Historically women have been underrepresented in clinical research, and diverse populations such as African Americans, Hispanics, Native Americans, and Asian/Pacific Islanders have been excluded. More research is needed looking at variables of HTN, diabetes, smoking, obesity, and the effect of a sedentary lifestyle across all ethnic populations [12].

Why the increase in incidence and prevalence of heart failure in women?

The incidence and prevalence of HF increase dramatically in women around the age of 65 years. HF rates are higher in women because women live longer with risk factors and post-MI sequelae, allowing time for HF to develop. As physicians become more aware of gender differences, and with advances in noninvasive diagnostic testing, medical management, and implementation of earlier percutaneous coronary intervention, women are more likely to receive an accurate diagnosis and efficacious treatment. Aggressive management can delay and/or prevent the development of HF in women who normally would have developed HF [7].

Classification and staging of heart failure

The New York Heart Association Classification of HF and the AHA/American College of

Cardiology staging of HF are outlined in Tables 1 and 2.

Clinical presentation

Women initially report warning signs of nausea, fatigue, dizziness, and shortness of breath but often do not see these symptoms as sufficient to seek prompt health care. Greater numbers of women seek medical care for symptoms of dyspnea and extreme fatigue. Health care providers sometimes mistake women's atypical symptoms as being musculoskeletal, gastrointestinal, or neurologic in origin instead of a cardiac problem [13].

Symptoms and diagnostic testing

The common signs and symptoms of HF are outlined in Box 3, and diagnostic testing in is outlined in Box 4.

2007 Updated Evidence-based Guidelines for Cardiovascular Disease Prevention in Women

The AHA updated the 2004 Guidelines for Cardiovascular Disease Prevention in Women. Primarily, the updated guidelines incorporate newer evidence with a focus on determining lifetime risk rather than short-term absolute risk. In the risk stratification assessment, the 2007 guidelines now categorize lifetime risk for women as "high risk," "at risk," and "optimal risk," with a primary focus on the prevention of heart

Table 1
New York Heart Association Functional Classification

Class	Patient symptoms
Class I: mild	No limitation in physical activity, and fatigue, palpitations, and dyspnea are absent.
Class II: mild	Slight limitation in physical activity. Patient is comfortable at rest but does experience fatigue, palpitation, or dyspnea.
Class III: moderate	Marked limitation in physical activity. Patient is comfortable at rest, but less than ordinary activity produces fatigue, palpitation, or dyspnea.
Class IV: severe	Patient cannot carry out any physical activity without discomfort. Activity increases discomfort level.

Table 2
American Heart Association/American College of Cardiology staging of heart failure

Stage	Definition	Examples
A	High risk for developing heart failure but no structural heart disorders	Hypertension, coronary artery disease Diabetes History of drug or alcohol abuse History of rheumatic fever Family history of cardiomyopathy
B	Structural heart disorders but no symptoms of heart failure	Left ventricular structural changes Valvular disease Myocardial infarction
C	Past or current symptoms of heart failure and underlying structural heart disease	Left ventricular systolic dysfunction with shortness of breath or fatigue Asymptomatic patient being treated for prior symptoms of heart failure
D	End-stage disease requiring specialized treatment strategies	Frequent hospitalizations for recurrent heart failure Patient unable to be discharged safely Patient awaiting heart transplant Patient at home but requiring intravenous therapy for relief of symptoms, support with mechanical assist devices Patient in hospice setting for management of heart failure

disease. Although there is growing consensus that the Framingham risk function has limitations for various populations of women, the Framingham Heart Study global risk scores still are used to guide lipid therapy [5].

Lipid management

Lipid levels can be reduced through lifestyle therapy, the use of statins to lower low-density lipoprotein (LDL) cholesterol levels, and the use

Box 3. Signs and symptoms of heart failure [14]

Early (mild impairment)
Difficulty breathing
Dyspnea on exertion (cardinal sign of left heart failure)
Tachypnea with mild exertion
Increased S3 heart sound
Basilar crackles
Nocturia
Diminishing functional capacity
Weakness and easily fatigues
Increased hepatojugular reflux

Moderate impairment
Two-pillow orthopnea
Paroxysmal nocturnal dyspnea
Anxiety
Wheezing
Tachypnea at rest
Nocturnal dry, hacking cough
Cardiomegaly
Increased S3, S4 sounds
Hypertension (diastolic)
Prominent bibasilar crackles
Right pleural effusion
Hepatomegaly with tenderness to palpation
Peripheral pitting edema
Peripheral vasoconstriction (cool extremities)

Severe impairment
Ascites
Anasarca
Hypotension
Frothy, pink sputum
Cyanosis
Cerebral dysfunction
Pulsus alternans
Cardiac cachexia
Cheyne-Stokes respirations

Data from Epocrates essentials. 2008. Available at: www.epocratesessentials.com. Accessed January 18, 2008.

Box 4. Diagnostic testing in heart failure

12-Lead EKG
Electrical conduction and ventricular enlargement

Chest radiograph
Pulmonary edema, cardiomegaly
Mild impairment: Increased heart size, increased blood flow to the upper lobes
Moderate severe impairment: Interstitial edema, Kerley's B lines, perivascular edema, sub-pleural effusions
Severe impairment: Alveolar edema, butterfly pattern of pulmonary edema

Echocardiogram
Measures ejection fraction, assesses valvular function.
Doppler ultrasound looks at blood flow through heart, pericardial effusion, identifies clot formation.

Cardiac catheterization
Evaluates coronary blockages, heart pressures, and cardiac output.

Exercise stress test
Tests exercise capacity and effects of exercise on the heart. Imaging stress test is more accurate than standard stress testing.

Brain natriuretic peptide
Differentiates heart failure from other medical conditions, such as lung involvement and/or determines degree of heart failure
B-type natriuretic peptide > 100 is a marker of ventricular dysfunction consistent with heart failure

Electrolytes
Assesses metabolic imbalances
Respiratory alkalosis, mild azotemia, decreased erythrocyte sedimentation rate, proteinuria usually < 1 g/24 hours, which clears with treatment
Dilutional hyponatremia, hyperbilirubinemia in severe heart failure

Blood urea nitrogen/creatinine levels
Creatinine levels are increased

Lipid profile
Assesses heart risk and determines treatment

of niacin or fibrate therapy for low HDL cholesterol or elevated non-HDL cholesterol levels after the target LDL cholesterol level is achieved. Treatment needs to occur when the LDL cholesterol is 190 mg/dL or higher, regardless of whether other risk factors are present [5]. According to the

AHA, lowering total cholesterol by 10% through early recognition and treatment of lipid levels may decrease the incidence of coronary heart disease by 30% [15].

Hormone replacement therapy and folic acid

Definitive data are integrated in the updated guidelines regarding the use of hormone replacement therapy, aspirin, and folic acid in postmenopausal women. Hormone replacement therapy and selective estrogen-receptor modulators, antioxidant supplements (vitamins E, C, and beta-carotene), and folic acid (with or without vitamin B_6 and B_{12}) are not suitable for primary or secondary prevention of cardiovascular heart disease. Data from the Heart and Estrogen/Progestin Replacement Study (HERS) and the HERS II follow-up revealed that most subjects had HFNEF, and hormone replacement therapy offered no survival benefit for women who had HF [16].

Aspirin

Aspirin is not cardioprotective in women until after age 65 years, but low-dose aspirin, 81 mg/d or 100 mg every other day, should be considered for stroke prevention in all women. In determining therapy, blood pressure must be controlled and the benefit must be weighed against the risk of gastrointestinal bleeding and hemorrhagic stroke.

The guidelines provide an algorithm to assist health care providers in prioritizing prevention interventions and evaluating the risk of cardiovascular disease in women [5].

How to manage heart failure

Immediate treatment of HF includes searching for an underlying modifiable condition and eliminating contributing factors, when possible. Initially patients are hospitalized, brain natriuretic peptide levels and laboratory values are obtained. They undergo diagnostic testing, then treated with supplemental oxygen, diuretics, fluid and sodium restrictions, low molecular weight heparin, and antiembolism stockings. Vital signs are checked frequently, along with telemetry and pulse oximetry monitoring. Weight is checked daily. During the severe stage, patients need bed rest with the head of the bed elevated. A gradual increase in activity by walking helps increase strength.

Patients move in and out of the various stages of HF throughout the course of the disease. Patient education plays a key role in the treatment of HF.

Unless contraindicated, preventive drugs as outlined in Table 3 should be used indefinitely after MI, with acute coronary syndrome, when the left ventricular ejection fraction (LVEF) is 40% or lower (with or without HF symptoms). Over-the-counter cough or cold medicines, ibuprofen, and naproxen should be avoided.

Educating patients to live a healthy life

Changing habits can be a daunting challenge for women who juggle multiple roles and responsibilities. Once women become aware of what is needed and make a commitment to bettering their condition, however, small changes can make a big difference in their attitude, long-term health, and benefit to their families. Women need to continue modifying their lifestyle and to add health-promoting behaviors.

In 2002, Krumholz and colleagues found that education and support alone decrease the rate of readmission and the cost of hospital stay. Nurses need to focus on the key components of patient education: activity, diet, medication, fluid consumption, weight monitoring, exercise, and signs and symptoms of worsening HF [2].

Smoking

If a patient is a smoker, she should stop. Patients also should avoid environmental smoke, which worsens HF. Nicotine replacements, pharmacologic agents, and smoking cessation programs are available to assist those wanting to quit smoking.

Weight

Being overweight adds strain on the heart muscle and makes breathing difficult. The patient should check her weight at the same time each morning after urination. She should use the same scale and document her weight in a monthly calendar log (Appendix 1).

Activity

A referral to a cardiac rehabilitation program should be considered to assist patients in increasing their activity levels while being monitored. The patient should talk with her physician before starting an exercise program. She should not exercise 1 to 2 hours after eating and should avoid exercising in extreme temperatures. She should start with slow, short walks of 5 minutes a day, 6 or 7 days a week. She should increase the walks gradually, adding 5 minutes each week. When tired, she should return to a lower level of activity for a few days. She should avoid lifting heavy objects or engaging in activities that cause dizziness, moderate shortness of breath, or chest discomfort. Sexual activity takes the same amount of energy as climbing one or two flights of stairs and may be resumed according to physician's instructions.

Diet

The patient should make an effort to choose foods high in whole-grain fiber, to add more fruits and vegetables, to limit sodium to 1 teaspoon per day, to reduce her intake of saturated fat and trans-fatty acids, to eat 12 ounces of fish each week, and to restrict her cholesterol intake to less than 300 mg/d. Patients need a formal dietary consultation. Box 5 lists high-sodium foods and offers suggestions for making healthful selections when dining out.

Alcohol consumption

Alcohol consumption should be limited to one drink per day, that is, 12 ounces of beer, 5 ounces of wine, or 1.5 ounces of 80-proof hard liquor.

Reading labels

The patient should pay attention to the serving size and the number of servings per container and compare those sizes with what actually is consumed. She should check the amount of sodium per serving and consume less than 2000 mg/d (< 1 teaspoon). Sodium is listed in the ingredients as salt, sodium, monosodium glutamate (MSG), baking soda/powder, or sodium chloride. The patient should be vigilant regarding foods labeled "reduced sodium" and select foods that contain 200 mg or less of sodium for one serving. She should look for foods labeled "salt-free," "sodium-free," or "low sodium."

Pneumonia/influenza

An annual flu vaccine and pneumococcal vaccine before age 65 years are recommended. The patient should avoid anyone who has a cold or flu and should stay away from crowds during the flu season.

Clothing and environment

The patient should avoid extreme hot or cold temperatures or wearing tightly fitted clothing and thigh-high or knee-high socks or stockings that reduce blood flow to the legs.

When to seek treatment

A patient should seek treatment when she observes

- A weight increase of 3 pounds in 1 day or more than 5 pounds a week
- Dizziness or shortness of breath while lying down or with any activity
- Edema in the ankles, feet, or legs that does not go away with elevation of the extremity
- A persistent cough, whether moist or dry
- A decrease in urination during the day with an increase in nocturia.
- Fatigue or loss of energy
- Side effects from medications, such as bradycardia less than 50 beats per minute, new onset of palpitations, chest pain, wheezing, skin rash, trouble swallowing, leg cramps, nausea/vomiting, or diarrhea.

Coping with chronic disease

HF is chronic and terminal, and coping with the condition can be difficult and stressful. Often individuals are not able to provide for their families or to participate in their usual activities, and as a result their social circles may dwindle. A person who has HF may require increasing assistance with activities of daily living. Financial concerns mount from a reduction in income, and the rising cost of medications and repeated hospitalizations over the course of the illness may place a tremendous burden on the family. With the stress resulting from dealing with chronic symptoms of end-stage cardiac disease, personal mortality, and the effect of the disease on significant others, fear and depression can occur.

Depression affects a patient's attitudes and outlook on life and the ability to function or to change lifestyle behaviors. Recognizing the signs and symptoms of depression is the first step. There may be feelings of sadness, worthlessness, trouble sleeping or concentrating, problems remembering things, feeling tired most of the time with no desire to engage in normal activities, or a weight loss or gain that cannot be explained. Women should be encouraged to reach out to family and friends for help or talk about feelings with a trusted person. Depression is more prevalent in women and increases the risk for first time and recurrent MIs.

Table 3
Medications used to treat heart failure

Type of medication	Examples of medications	Mechanism of action	Indications	Administration	Possible reactions/side effects	Precautions (nursing considerations)
Beta-blockers (name ends in "olol")	Atenolol (Tenormin) Carvedilol (Coreg) Metoprolol (Lopressor, Toprol XL) Propanolol (Inderal) Sotalol (Betapace) Labetalol (Normodyne) Nadolol (Corgard)	Blocks beta receptors in the heart to decrease workload of the heart and myocardial oxygen demand by lowering heart rate, force of contraction, and rate of A-V conduction Decreases myocardial injury during MI and can lessen scarring of heart muscle following MI	Angina Hypertension Heart failure Prevent second MI Prevent and treat irregular heart rate: SVT, PVCs Migraines	Take apical pulse for full minute before dose. Document. Call doctor if heart rate <60 bpm. Give with food Do not discontinue abruptly, can exacerbate angina or precipitate MI (over 3 days to 2 weeks)	☑ Bradycardia or heart blocks ☑ Hypotension ☑ Bronchospasms ☑ Numbness/ tingling/ cold in hands and feet ☑ Lethargy ☑ Depression ☑ Heart failure ☑ Gastrointestinal disturbance ☑ Sexual dysfunction ☑ Watch diabetic patients for sweating, fatigue, hunger, because signs of hypoglycemia may be masked	Monitor and document apical heart rate, blood pressure, and EKG rhythm Elderly patients and patients with renal and liver failure need adjusted doses Watch drug interactions with digoxin and calcium-channel blockers, because both decrease conduction and with diuretics, which decrease blood pressure Contraindications: ◎ Sinus bradycardia or heart blocks ◎ Patients who have asthma or COPD may develop bronchospasms ◎ Decompensated heart failure Antidote: Intravenous atropine or glucagon reverses beta-blocker overdose

Class	Drugs	Action	Uses	Administration	Adverse reactions	Nursing considerations
Angiotensin-converting enzyme inhibitors (name ends in "pril")	Captopril (Capoten) Enalapril (Vasotec) Fosinopril (Monopril) Ramipril (Altace) Benzaepril (Lotensin) Lisinopril (Prinivil, Zestril) Perindopril (Aceon) Trandolapril (Mavik) Quinapril (Accupril) Moexipril (Univase)	Blocks angiotensin II (potent vasoconstrictor responsible for increasing blood pressure) to lower blood pressure and decrease peripheral vascular resistance	Hypertension Heart failure (ejection fraction < 35%–40%), post MI Increases survival in heart failure, MI, and stroke Can protect diabetic patients from developing kidney disease	Usually given once a day, 1 hour before meals	☑ First dose: hypotension ☑ Dry persistent cough ☑ Dizziness ☑ Tachycardia ☑ Orthostatic hypotension ☑ Gastrointestinal distress ☑ Headache ☑ Increased potassium levels ☑ Can worsen kidney function Oliguria or progressive azotemia	Check blood pressure and heart rate before and after administration Watch for excessive hypotension in patients taking diuretics Monitor urine output Caution: Serum creatinine > 3 mg/dL or creatinine clearance < 30 mL/min (half dosage) Autoimmune diseases (SLE) Contraindications: ◎ Intolerance to angiotensin-converting enzyme inhibitors ◎ Potassium level > 5.5mEq/L that cannot be reduced ◎ Symptomatic hypotension
Diuretics Loop	Furosemide (Lasix) Bumetanide (Bumex) Ethacrynic acid (Edecrin)	Inhibits absorption of sodium, chlorine, and potassium in the loop of Henle Rapid onset, short duration High ceiling	Hypertension Heart failure Pulmonary and peripheral edema Ascites	Give in morning to prevent nocturia Pulmonary edema requires intravenous administration dose to be given	☑ Dehydration ☑ Hypotension ☑ Ototoxicity (hearing loss) ☑ Elevated serum urea nitrogen ☑ Dizziness, vertigo, headache, blurred vision	Monitor blood pressure, heart rate, intake and output, weight Monitor serum electrolytes, potassium, magnesium Monitor serum urea nitrogen/creatinine Watch for orthostatic hypotension, tachycardia, poor skin turgor, and excessive thirst Add potassium-rich foods

(continued on next page)

Table 3 (continued)

Type of medication	Examples of medications	Mechanism of action	Indications	Administration	Possible reactions/side effects	Precautions (nursing considerations)
Thiazide	Hydrochlorothiazide (HydroDiuril)	Increases sodium, chlorine, and water excretion in proximal portion of distal tubule	Hypertension Mild to moderate heart failure Peripheral edema Nephrotic syndrome Cirrhosis	Give in morning	☑ Hyperglycemia in diabetic patients ☑ Dehydration ☑ Elevated uric acid levels (gout) ☑ Decreases potassium and magnesium levels	Monitor serum electrolytes Monitor blood pressure, heart rate, intake and output, weight May need potassium supplements Monitor serum urea nitrogen/creatinine Check blood glucose levels in diabetic patients
Potassium-sparing	Amiloride (Midamor) Spironolactone (Aldactone) Triamterene (Dyrenium)	Aldosterone blocker in distal convoluted tubule to retain potassium and excrete sodium	Hypertension Edema Diuretic-induced hypokalemia in patients who have heart failure Renovascular Hypertension	Give with meals	☑ Muscle cramps ☑ Increased potassium levels with development of lethal arrhythmia ☑ Elevated serum urea nitrogen	Monitor EKG for PVC arrhythmias Monitor blood pressure, heart rate, intake and output, weight Monitor serum electrolytes Caution: Renal impairment Patients also receiving angiotensin-converting enzyme inhibitors Increases the half-life of digoxin Contraindications: ◎ Renal failure ◎ High potassium levels

Abbreviations: A-V, Atrial Ventricular; COPD, chronic obstructive pulmonary disease; MI, myocardial infarction; PVC, premature ventricular contractions; SLE, systemic lupus erythematosus; SVT, supraventricular tachycardia.

Courtesy of Angela Pruitt, MSN, RN, CNS, Evansville, IN.

Box 5. High-sodium foods

High-sodium foods to avoid
  Bacon, ham, sausage
  Smoked or dried meat, chicken or fish; chipped beef; corned beef; tuna packed in oil
  Canned meat, fish, chicken, vegetables, soups, stews, or dinners
  Hotdogs, bologna, salami, and cold cuts
  Instant, processed foods
  "Fast" foods
  Pickles, relish, olives
  Sauces: Worcestershire sauce, steak, chili, barbecue, cocktail, teriyaki
  Snack foods: potato or corn chips, pretzels, nuts
  Seasonings: onion salt, garlic salt, celery salt, and bouillon
  Chinese foods

Dining outside the home
  Select baked, broiled, or grilled entrées
  Choose baked or boiled potatoes, plain rice or pasta, and whole-grain breads
  Select fresh fruit, juice, or salad with oil and vinegar dressing
  Order salad dressing on the side
  Avoid foods prepared with gravy, soy sauce, or monosodium glutamate (MSG)
  Do not add salt to food at the table
  Avoid olives, pickles, croutons, cheese, bacon bits, mayonnaise, and marinated
    or cream-based salads
  Desserts: choose fresh fruit, fruit ice, gelatin, fruit salad, or angel food cake

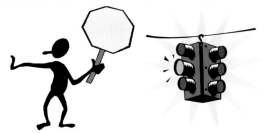

Health care professionals should encourage women to be their own advocates in requesting referrals or treatment with selective serotonin reuptake inhibitors [5].

Caregivers are affected by the increased or new responsibilities and often forego personal interests because of lack of time and energy. It is equally important for the caregiver to stay healthy, to get plenty of rest, and to eat a balanced diet. Exercising and accepting offers of help from others can assist in stress reduction. Emotional balance is maintained better when the caregiver is able to communicate feelings to the patient who has HF and/or family members and stay involved in activities he or she enjoys.

Social services are a valuable resource in finding support for caring for a person who has HF. Services may include meal delivery, errand services, transportation, home health agencies, prescription delivery, support groups, or churches and volunteer centers willing to provide a respite from the daily care.

How do we improve heart failure education for women?

Health care providers need to supply HF education in written format. Many hospitals are creating educational booklets on HF for distribution to patients at discharge. Topics covered include definitions of terms, information on how the heart works, causes of and risk factors for HF, signs and symptoms of HF, testing and treatments for HF, diet, activity, and what to do when patients get home. A medication list (Appendix 2) and a monthly chart for recording daily weights and symptoms assist patients who have HF in identifying a trend of worsening symptoms.

Nurses

Nurses may be contributing to noncompliance and readmissions by not providing adequate education to patients and their families. Washburn and colleagues [2] studied nurses' knowledge of HF education topics and found that both intensive care and floor nurses are unaware deficiencies exist in their knowledge of HF and what to teach patients.

Nurses are central in the education of patients and need to be able to recognize their own deficiencies in knowledge and assume responsibility for obtaining the essential information so they can teach patients how to manage end-stage cardiac disease. This crucial knowledge enhances the patient's ability to self-manage HF and improves the patient's quality of life.

Health care practices continue to change, and the fast-paced environment affects nursing practice. Status quo no longer exists, and nurses must be involved in and have current knowledge about evidence-based practice. As nurses assume ownership of their nursing practice, the quality of patient care improves. Hospital administrators and clinical educators need to ensure that funding and opportunities are available for nurses' continuing education, including both didactic and clinical experiences.

A multidisciplinary approach becomes essential to reduce readmissions, length of stay, and cost of care. Advanced nurse practitioners can be leaders in care conferences, addressing and individualizing the needs of patients before discharge, and can serve as liaison with physicians, nurses, and patients.

Health care providers must offer avenues to educate the public about the atypical symptoms women experience, because 36% of women do not consider themselves to be at risk for coronary heart disease. Nursing can take the lead in providing community education to influence women's health through health fairs, formal and informal education programs, clinics, screenings, and providing brochures and pamphlets to churches, schools, and women's clubs. Community venues serve to increase the knowledge bout HF in women and the effect of heart disease within the community [12].

Physicians

A large percentage of physicians still are unaware that an increasing number of women die each year from heart disease. Educational efforts are needed in medical and nursing schools to integrate current guidelines and practices for HF in women [15].

Physicians must take notice that 25% of women stated that their health care providers did not communicate the importance of heart health, and one woman in five reported her health care provider did not explain clearly how to change her risk status [5]. All health care providers must improve the quality of their communication. They must allow time to address a patient's questions, offer practical information, and ensure the patient understands her risk of HF or the medical care required for management of HF [5].

Society

The media has disseminated mixed messages about hormone replacement therapy and aspirin therapy and has not publicized adequately the information that each year more women die from heart disease than from all forms of cancer combined [5].

Women need to know they do report more symptoms than men and should no longer fear being labeled a hypochondriac. Women must take the time and responsibility for managing their own health, not just the health of their family members. To change attitudes in women and caregivers, education needs to focus on explaining how health-promoting behaviors prevent heart disease and how HTN, diabetes, and obesity increase women's risk of heart disease [13].

Summary

Women require pharmacologic treatment with beta-blockers, angiotensin-converting enzyme inhibitors, and/or angiotensin-receptor blockers with a diuretic to symptomatically treat HF or control HTN. Nurses need to notice atypical and subtle changes as patients move between the various stages of HF. Early recognition of worsening HF symptoms and prompt medical treatment can minimize damage to the myocardium.

For women to be proactive, nurses need to advise patients to seek treatment when they experience a weight increase, shortness of breath, wheezing, dizziness, edema, persistent cough, nocturia, fatigue, bradycardia, chest pain, or palpitations. HF education booklets can serve as references for self-management and monitoring of symptoms at home.

Nurses continue to play a key role in patient education and need to seek continuing educational opportunities to stay current with evidence-based practice. All health care providers must provide opportunities for quality communication, allowing time to address patients' questions and ensure patients' adequate understanding of medical treatment.

Educational efforts in medical and nursing schools to integrate current guidelines and practices for women and HF will minimize the mixed messages women receive.

Appendix 1

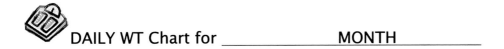 DAILY WT Chart for _____ MONTH _____

Monday	Tuesday	Wednesday	Thursday	Friday	Saturday	Sunday
Date: Wt: Symptoms:	Date: Wt: Symptoms:	Date: Wt: Symptoms:	Date: Wt: Symptoms:	Date: Wt: Symptoms:	Date: Wt: Symptoms:	Date: Wt: Symptoms:
Date: Wt: Symptoms:	Date: Wt: Symptoms:	Date: Wt: Symptoms:	Date: Wt: Symptoms:	Date: Wt: Symptoms:	Date: Wt: Symptoms:	Date: Wt: Symptoms:
Date: Wt: Symptoms:	Date: Wt: Symptoms:	Date: Wt: Symptoms:	Date: Wt: Symptoms:	Date: Wt: Symptoms:	Date: Wt: Symptoms:	Date: Wt: Symptoms:
Date: Wt: Symptoms:	Date: Wt: Symptoms:	Date: Wt: Symptoms:	Date: Wt: Symptoms:	Date: Wt: Symptoms:	Date: Wt: Symptoms:	Date: Wt: Symptoms:

Symptoms:

A. Loss of appetite or nausea
B. Tired
C. Cough or chest congestion
D. Restless
E. Swelling legs, feet, hands, abdomen

F. Increase shortness of breath with activity
G. Sleeping with more pillows than usual
H. Dizzy or lightheaded
I. Fast heart beat
J. Bubbly sputum

Rate your Symptoms on Scale: 1-2-3-4-5
1 = Mild; 3 = Moderate; 5 = Severe

REMEMBER: Weigh yourself at the <u>same time</u>, in the same <u>clothing</u> every day, using the same <u>scales</u>. Notify your doctor if you have a sudden weight gain of **3 pounds per day,** or more than **5 pounds a week**. Take this sheet with you to all doctor appointments.

Appendix 2

MEDICINE LIST for _____

Name of Medicine	Amount	Reason for Taking	6 a m	8 a m	10 a m	12 Noon	2p m	4 p m	6 p m	8 p m	10 p m	12 M N	Special Direction

Resources for heart failure

The American Heart Association: www. americanheart.org
Heart Failure Society of America www.hfsa.org
About Heart Failure: www.abouthf.org/

National Heart Blood and Lung Institute www.nhlbi.nih.gov/
National Institute on Aging www.nia.nih.gov
Cleveland Clinic Heart & Vascular Institute http://www.clevelandclinic.org/heartcenter/pub/guide/disease/heartfailure.asp?firstCat=3&secondCat=246&thirdCat=256

Mayo Clinic http://www.mayoclinic.com/health/heart-failure/DS00061

U.S. Food and Drug Administration http://www.fda.gov/hearthealth/conditions/congestiveheartfailure.html

Texas Heart Institute http://www.texasheartinstitute.org/HIC/Topics/Cond/CHF.cfm

Center for Disease Control and Prevention http://www.cdc.gov/dhdsp/library/fs_heart_failure.htm

CAREGIVERS

The National Family Caregivers Association http://www.familycaregiving101.org/

The Heart of Caregiving http://www.americanheart.org/presenter.jhtml?identifier=3039829

Heartmates: Resources For The Spouse, Family, and Loved Ones of a Heart Patient: http://www.heartmates.com/

Well Spouse Association: Support for Spousal Caregivers http://www.wellspouse.org/

The American Association of Retired Persons (AARP) http://www.aarp.org

Administration on Aging, US Department of Health and Human Services, http://www.aoa.gov

Today's Caregiver Magazine http://www.caregiver.com

References

[1] Sandmaier M. NIH Publication No. 07–2720. National Institutes of Health; 2007.

[2] Washburn S, Hornberger C, Klutman A, et al. Nurses' knowledge of heart failure education topics as reported in a small Midwestern community hospital. J Cardiovasc Nurs 2005;20(3):215–20.

[3] Owan T, Hodge D, Herges R, et al. Trends in prevalence and outcome of heart failure with preserved ejection fraction. N Engl J Med 2006;355(3):251–9. Available at: http://content.nejm.org/cgi/content/full/355/3/251?ijkey=2980a6ae62420a34888fd7a1bebc0986b99bd727. Accessed November 17, 2007.

[4] American Heart Association. Available at: http://circ.ahajournals.org/cgi/content/fullCIRCULATIONAHA.106.179918#TBL1179733. Accessed January 14, 2008.

[5] Mosca L, Banka CL, Benjamin EJ, et al. Evidence-based guidelines for cardiovascular disease prevention in women: 2007 update. Circulation 2007;115(11):1481–501.

[6] Heart disease and stroke statistics 2008 update. A report from the American Heart Association Statistics Committee and Stroke Statistics Subcommittee. Circulation Journal of the American Heart Association. Available at: http://circ.ahajournals.org/cgi/reprint/CIRCULATIONAHA.107.187998v1. Accessed January 14, 2008.

[7] Lund L, Mancini D. Heart failure in women. Med Clin North Am 2004;88(5):1321–45.

[8] Women's Health Initiative. Available at: http://www.nhlbi.nih.gov/whi/factsht.htm. Accessed January 12, 2008.

[9] Heart disease and stroke statistics. 2008 update at a glance. Available at: http://www.americanheart.org/downloadable/heart/1198257493273HS_Stats%202008.pdf. Accessed January 14, 2008.

[10] Hsia J, Margolis K, Eaton C, et al. Prehypertension and cardiovascular disease risk in the Women's Health Initiative. Circulation 2007;115:855–60.

[11] Matthews KA, Sowers MF, Derby CA, et al. Ethnic differences in cardiovascular risk factor burden among middle-aged women: Study of Women's Health Across the Nation (SWAN). Am Heart J 2005;149(6):1066–73.

[12] Hart P. Women's perceptions of coronary heart disease: an integrative review. J Cardiovasc Nurs 2005;20(3):170–6 [OVID Full Text].

[13] Patel H, Rosengren A, Ekman I. Symptoms in acute coronary syndromes: does sex make a difference? Am Heart J 2004;148(1):27–33.

[14] Epocrates essentials. 2008. Available at: www.epocratesessentials.com. Accessed January 18, 2008.

[15] Trynosky K. Missed targets: gender differences in the identification and management of dyslipidemia. J Cardiovasc Nurs 2006;21(5):342–6.

[16] Bibbins-Domingo K, Lin F, Vittinghoff E, et al. Effect of hormone therapy on mortality rates among women with heart failure and coronary artery disease. Am J Cardiol 2005;95(2):289–91.

ELSEVIER
SAUNDERS

Crit Care Nurs Clin N Am 20 (2008) 343–350

CRITICAL CARE
NURSING CLINICS
OF NORTH AMERICA

Chemotherapy-Induced Cardiotoxicity in Women

Kelli S. Dempsey, MSN, APRN-BC, AOCNP

American Cancercare, 2613 E. Walnut Street, Evansville, IN 47714, USA

Chemotherapy-induced cardiotoxicity (CIC) can cause treatment dilemmas, decreased survival, increased morbidity, and complicated psychosocial issues. The purpose of this article is threefold: to define CIC; to discuss a model for evaluation and treatment; and to present a case study.

Heart disease is the leading cause of death in the United States, with cancer a very close second. The American Cancer Society estimates that 678,060 women were diagnosed with cancer and 270,100 women died of cancer in the United States during 2007. The three most common sites of cancer in women are breast (26%), lung (15%), and colon (11%) [1]. Every 3 minutes a women in the United States is diagnosed with breast cancer [2]. In 2007, more than 176,000 women were diagnosed with breast cancer, and more than 40,000 in the United States died of this disease [1]. The incidence of breast cancer in women has increased from 1 in 20 in 1960 to one in eight in 2007 [2]. Although CIC is not unique to women, some of the most common cardiotoxic agents are chemotherapy drugs used to treat breast cancer. In the United States, 99% of patients who have breast cancer are female [3]. Therefore the scope of this article is limited to CIC in women who have breast cancer.

The median age for women at diagnosis of breast cancer is 61 years, and the median age of death caused by breast cancer is 69 years. The overall 5-year survival rate for women who have breast cancer is 88%. In 2004, there were more than 2 million women alive in the United States who had a history of breast cancer [4]. Improvements in the detection and treatment of breast cancer have resulted in a 24% decrease in mortality from breast cancer since 1990 [5]. Breast cancer is becoming a manageable chronic disease, comparable in its chronicity to diabetes or hypertension [6]. Many survivors of breast cancer actually are at greater risk of death from cardiovascular disease than from cancer [6].

Chemotherapy-induced cardiotoxicity

Cardiotoxicity is defined as a poisonous or deleterious effect upon the heart [7]. CIC is cardiotoxicity that develops as a result of chemotherapy administration. CIC can manifest on a continuum ranging from asymptomatic, transient arrhythmias to fatal cardiomyopathy resulting from permanent left ventricular dysfunction. CIC may occur acutely during treatment or years later and varies for different chemotherapy drugs [8]. Table 1 summarizes the cardiotoxic manifestations of various chemotherapy drugs, and Box 1 offers related definitions.

The signs and symptoms of cardiotoxicity vary widely. Signs of cardiac dysfunction may include changes in blood pressure or heart rate, irregular heart rhythms, murmurs, carotid bruits, distended jugular veins, decreased pulses, edema, and changes in skin color [9]. The most common symptoms of cardiac problems associated with cardiotoxicity are pain, dyspnea, weight gain, edema, weakness, fatigue, palpitations, dizziness, syncope and swelling of an extremity with deep venous thromboembolism [10].

The quality of pain varies with the cardiac disorder present. Ischemic pain often presents as pressing, squeezing, or a weight-like pressure on the chest and possibly radiating to the neck, arm, or jaw. Pericardial inflammatory pain feels like burning or stabbing and worsens with coughing or lying down. Pulmonary embolism pain typically is pleuritic and usually is associated with dyspnea [10]. Dyspnea is uncomfortable or

E-mail address: kellidempsey@insightbb.com

0899-5885/08/$ - see front matter © 2008 Elsevier Inc. All rights reserved.
doi:10.1016/j.ccell.2008.03.004

Table 1
Chemotherapy agents associated with cardiotoxicity

Condition	Chemotherapeutic Agent
Angina	Cytarabine; fludarabine
Arrhythmias	All-trans retinoic acid (ATRA); arsenic trioxide; aldesleukin; busulfan (tamponade); capecitabine; cisplatin; cyclophosphamide (high dose);cytarabine; daunorubicin (acute); dimethyl sulfoxide; doxorubicin (acute); epirubicin (acute); fluorouracil; idarubicin (acute); ifosfamide; interferons; decitabine; methotrexate; mitoxantrone; paclitaxel; rituximab; thalidomide
Cardiogenic shock	Fluorouracil
Cardiomyopathy	Cyclophosphamide; daunorubicin; epirubicin (chronic); trastuzumab
Chronic heart failure	Aldesleukin; ATRA; alemtuzumab (chronic); bevacizumab; capecitabine; cisplatin; cytarabine; daunorubicin (chronic); decitabine; doxorubicin (chronic); epirubicin (chronic); fluorouracil; idarubicin (chronic); ifofsamide; imatinib; interferon (high-dose); mitomycin; mitoxantrone; paclitaxel; pentostatin; trastuzumab
Deep venous thromboembolism	Bevacizumab; thalidomide
Edema	Imatinib; thalidomide
Effusion	ATRA; imatinib
Endomyocardial fibrosis	Busulfan
Heart block	Cyclophosphamide; cisplatin; interferon
Hypertension	Bevacizumab; bleomycin; cisplatin; mitomycin; procarbazine; vinblastine
Hypotension	Aldesleukin; alemtuzumab; ATRA; carmustine; cetuximab dacarbazine; denileukin diftitox; etoposide; fludarabine; interferon; paclitaxel; rituximab; tamoxifen; thalidomide; vincristine
Ischemia/infarction	ATRA; bevacizumab; bleomycin; capecitabine; cisplatin; dactinomycin; epirubicin (chronic); etoposide
Left ventricular dysfunction	Interferon; trastuzumab
Myocarditis/pericarditis	ATRA; bleomycin; cyclophosphamide; cytarabine; doxorubicin; etoposide; mitoxantrone
Possible cardiac toxicity	Altretamine; amifostine; aminoglutethimide; anagrelide; anastrazole; bevacizumab; bexarotene; campath; cytarabine (liposomal); estramustine; etoposide; exemestane; flutamide; gosrelin; leuprolide; megesterol acetate; oprelvekin; oxaliplatin; tamoxifen; teniposide; thalidomide; tretinoin
Vasospasm	Interferon; trastuzumab

From: Mays, Theresa. 2007 Oncology Preparatory Review Course Handbook. Used with permission from the American College of Clinical Pharmacy and the American Society of Health-System Pharmacists; with permission.

labored breathing which worsens with exertion and when lying down. Palpitations are the perception of heart action and may be associated with increased weakness, fatigue, and dizziness [10]. Patients receiving potentially cardiotoxic chemotherapy agents and their family members/caregivers should be educated about the signs and symptoms of cardiotoxicities and about the need to notify health care personnel when signs or symptoms of these conditions occur.

Model of evaluation and treatment

Evaluation

The general model for the evaluation and treatment of CIC is similar to that used to evaluate and design treatment regimens for patients who have breast cancer. An oncologist typically is consulted to see a patient who has a known diagnosis of breast cancer, often after biopsy and/or surgical intervention. To help guide prognosis and treatment choices, the oncology evaluation includes determination of the stage, grade, hormone receptor, and HER2 status of the tumor [11].

The treatment and prognosis of breast cancer depend on staging (extent of cancer) and tumor grade (pathologic features) [12,13]. Staging tests determine whether the cancer is invasive or noninvasive, the size of the tumor, lymph node involvement, and whether there is distant spread (metastasis). Stages range from 0 to 4. The percentage of patients at diagnosis and the 5-year survival rates vary for the different stages of breast cancer (Table 2) [4,12].

Staging of breast cancer uses history, examination, surgery, imaging, and laboratory tests. Surgical interventions after initial biopsy may include lumpectomy, mastectomy, axillary dissection, sentinel lymph node biopsy, and biopsy at site of metastasis [2,11]. Imaging techniques for staging include radiography, CT scan, bone scan, MRI, and PET scans [11]. Laboratory testing with blood cell counts, chemistry panels, and tumor markers provides information on the patient's overall health and organ

Table 2
The percentage of patients at diagnosis and the associated 5-year survival rates for the stages of breast cancer

Stage	Diagnosis (%)	5-year Survival (%)
0 and 1 (localized)	61	98
2 (local spread)	31 (combined with stage 3)	81–92
3 (locally advanced)	31	54–67
4 (distant spread)	6	20–26

function and helps identify areas of possible metastasis, such as bone or liver [11].

Once the need for treatment with chemotherapy, radiation, biologic, and/or hormonal therapy has been determined, evaluation for the patient's risk of developing CIC is indicated. Women who have breast cancer may have greater risk of developing cardiovascular disease because of risks associated with treatment as well as their prediagnosis risk stratification [14]. Women considering chemotherapy and/or hormone treatment after surgery and/or radiation therapy should be evaluated for pre-existing cardiovascular risk factors. These evaluations include the assessment of both modifiable and nonmodifiable risks. Modifiable risks (hyperlipidemia, smoking, sedentary lifestyle, high-caloric and/or high-fat diet, obesity, stress, hypertension, diabetes) and nonmodifiable risks (race, genetics, aging) should be assessed [15].

Researchers from Duke University Medical Center recommend performing a formal cardiovascular risk assessment, using either the Framingham or Reynolds risk scores on all patients who have breast cancer before initiation of chemotherapy or hormonal therapy [14]. The Framingham Heart Study prediction score takes into account age, high- and low-density cholesterol levels, blood pressure, smoking, and diabetes [16]. The Reynolds risk score considers age, smoking, systolic blood pressure, total and high-density cholesterol levels, C-reactive protein level, and parental history of myocardial infarction [17].

Treatment

The chemotherapy and biologic therapy agents most commonly used for breast cancer are listed in Table 3 along with their associated cardiotoxicities. The most common cardiotoxic agents are the anthracyclines (eg, doxorubicin and epirubicin) and the biologic agent, trastuzumab [8,22]. The incidence of clinical heart failure caused by anthracyclines is between 1% and 5% with

Table 3
Cardiotoxicity of chemotherapeutic agents used to treat breast cancer - synthesis of the literature [18,19,20,21]

Generic name	Brand name	Cardiotoxicity
Albumin-bound paclitaxel	Abraxane	None significant
Aromatase inhibitors	Arimidex, Aromasin, Faslodex, Femara	Angina, hypertension, infarction, thromboembolism
Bevacizumab	Avastin	Hypertension Ischemia Congestive heart failure
Capecitabine	Xeloda	Angina Congestive heart failure Ischemia
Carboplatin	Paraplatin	Ischemia
Cyclophosphamide	Cytoxan	Cardiomyopathy Myocarditis
Docetaxel	Taxotere	Edema
Doxorubicin	Adriamycin	See text
Epirubicin	Ellence	Arrhythmias Cardiomyopathy Congestive heart failure Ischemia
Fluorouracil	5-FU	Arrhythmias Congestive heart failure Ischemia
Gemcitabine	Gemzar	None significant
Lapatinib	Tykerb	Prolonged QT Decreased left ventricular ejection fraction
Methotrexate	Trexall	Arrhythmias Ischemia
Tamoxifen	Nolvadex	Thromboembolism
Trastuzumab	Herceptin	See text
Paclitaxel	Taxol	Arrhythmias Congestive heart failure Hypotension Ischemia
Pegylated liposomal doxorubicin	Doxil	CHF (must be included in measuring accumulated dose of athracycline)
Vinorelbine	Navelbine	Ischemia

asymptomatic decrease in left ventricular function ranging from 5% to 20%. Clinical heart failure increases when cardiotoxic drugs are used in combination [23].

Doxorubicin is the major chemotherapy agent used for treating breast cancer [24]. Cardiotoxicity associated with doxorubicin ranges from early-onset sinus tachycardia to late-onset fatal cardiomyopathy [8]. Acute toxicities include arrhythmias, pericarditis, myocardial infarction, sudden cardiac death, congestive heart failure (CHF), and cardiomyopathy [25]. Chronic toxicity with anthracyclines includes cardiomyopathy and CHF [25].

According to the Food and Drug Administration (FDA), a "black box" warning in the package insert alerts prescribers to the following serious potential problems [26]:

- An adverse reaction so serious in proportion to the potential benefit from the drug that it must be considered in assessing the risks and benefits of using the drug
- A serious adverse reaction that can be reduced or prevented
- FDA approval of drug that included restrictions to ensure safety

The doxorubicin package insert contains a black box warning regarding "myocardial toxicity manifested in its most severe form by potentially fatal CHF," which may occur during treatment or months to years after treatment [8].

Doxorubicin cardiotoxicity is related to the cumulative dosage a patient receives. The risk of cardiotoxicity ranges from 1% to 20% for doses of 300 mg/m^2 to 500 mg/m^2 [8]. Doxorubicin cardiotoxicity also varies with the route of administration. Intravenous push (IVP) administration involves drug delivery over a matter of minutes. Continuous infusion, however, entails intravenous delivery of medication over a 48- or 96-hour time period. Findings from a landmark study published in 1989 involving 141 patients showed a 75% decrease in clinical CHF when patients received doxorubicin by continuous infusion as compared with IVP. Although this study demonstrated that administration of doxorubicin by continuous infusion decreased cardiotoxicity, this slower method of drug delivery did not affect treatment response rate, time to response, duration of response, or survival [27].

Factors increasing the risk for anthracycline cardiotoxicity include prior mediastinal radiation, concurrent treatment with other cardiotoxic drugs, doxorubicin exposure at an early age, advanced patient age, and pre-existing heart disease [8]. A popular breast cancer regimen gives doxorubicin and cyclophosphamide for four cycles followed by paclitaxel with or without trastuzumab for four cycles [24]. Sequential administration of these drugs reduces cardiotoxicity [22,24].

Cardiac monitoring is crucial for all women starting treatment with an anthracycline. The baseline ejection fraction should be determined with either a multigated radionuclide angiography (MUGA) or echocardiography (ECHO) study [8]. Clinical monitoring by history and examination is mandatory to find symptoms and signs of heart problems. ECHO or MUGA is desirable at intervals during and after treatment [8]. Using the same technique for monitoring heart function provides consistency and improves recognition of deterioration in cardiac function [8].

The doxorubicin package insert defines deterioration of cardiac function by left ventricular ejection fraction (LVEF) measurement as a 10% decline below the lower limit of normal (50%–70%), an LVEF of 45% or less, or a 20% decline from the baseline LVEF [8]. When CIC occurs, the benefit of further treatment must be weighed against the risk of developing irreversible cardiac damage [8].

Her-2/Neu (HER2) is a gene that helps control cellular growth, division, repair, and helps control abnormal or defective cells [28]. The overamplification of *HER2* on a cell surface is thought to lead to increased cellular proliferation that can cause malignancy [29]. *HER2* is a poor prognostic indicator amplified in up to 30% of breast cancers and is associated with an increased risk of recurrence and death, increased incidence of positive lymph nodes, a 50% increased chance of brain metastases, and decreased response to hormonal therapy [30,31]. Conversely, *HER2*-positive breast cancers have a better response to anthracycline chemotherapy and thus have a better clinical prognosis [32].

Trastuzumab is a monoclonal antibody biologic therapy that is effective in *Her2*-positive tumors. A monoclonal antibody is a type of protein synthesized in the laboratory that locates and binds to specific receptors in the body and on the surface of cancer cells [28]. Two studies enrolling more than 3000 patients showed a dramatic reduction of up to 52% in overall risk of recurrence in early invasive breast cancer with the addition of trastuzumab to the chemotherapy regimen [33]. The increased risk of CHF from adding trastuzumab to chemotherapy was approximately 4%, a risk most patients are willing to assume for the added benefit [33].

Most women developing CHF (68%) had resolution of symptoms by 6 months after completion of trastuzumab treatment [33].

Trastuzumab includes a black box warning on the package insert regarding cardiomyopathy. The package insert notes that trastuzumab administration can result in left ventricular dysfunction and CHF, especially when administered with anthracyclines. Recommendations for decreasing the risk of CIC and improving detection of CIC include LVEF evaluation by ECHO or MUGA before beginning chemotherapy and frequently during treatment [22]. The large studies mentioned previously checked LVEF at baseline and at 3, 6, 9, 15, and 18 months [33]. Trastuzumab should be withheld or discontinued if there is a 16% or larger decrease from the baseline LVEF, an LVEF below normal with a 10% or greater decrease from baseline, persistent decreased LVEF for 8 weeks, and/or dosing interruptions on more than three occasions [22].

Adjuvantonline.com is an excellent Web-based resource that stratifies the risks and benefits of various treatments for breast, lung, and colon cancer. This resource includes a slide presentation from the 2005 meeting of the American Society of Clinical Oncology that shows a table describing pretreatment LVEF values, patient age, and subsequent risk of developing cardiomyopathy with trastuzumab treatment. For women under age 50 years, the risk for developing CHF for baseline a LVEF of 50% to 54% was reported to be 6.3%, compared with 19.1% for women older than 50 years. A baseline LVEF higher than 65% decreased the risk of developing CHF to 0.6% for women younger than 50 years and 1.3% for women older than 50 years.

Bevacizumab is a monoclonal antibody used to treat breast, colon, and lung cancer. The package insert contains a black box warning for gastrointestinal perforation, wound-healing complications, and pulmonary hemorrhage [34]. The package insert states that 1.7% of patients in the manufacturer's clinical studies developed CHF [34]. When used in patients who had prior or concurrent anthracycline use and/or left chest wall radiation, the incidence increased to 4% [34]. Bevacizumab use is associated with arterial thromboembolic events (VTE) and hypertension [34].

Thromboembolic events included stroke, transient ischemic attack (mini-stroke), myocardial infarction, and angina. Hypertension (> 150/100 mm Hg) and severe hypertension (> 200/110 mm Hg) were noted in as many as 18% of patients in clinical trials using bevacizumab. Patients treated with bevacizumab in oncology practices commonly develop hypertension that is manageable using antihypertensives [34]. The bevacizumab package insert recommends discontinuing or holding treatment until hypertension can be controlled [34].

Thromboembolism affects approximately 15% of all patients who have cancer (personal communication, A. Kommareddy, 2007). Combined with smoking, implanted venous access devices, and chemotherapy agents that increase the risk of clotting, thromboembolism becomes a significant issue. Hormonal therapy with tamoxifen and aromatase inhibitors has improved breast cancer survival [35,36]. Tamoxifen has a black box warning for VTE including stroke, deep venous thromboembolism, infarction, and fatal pulmonary embolism [35]. The risk for developing VTE is present, but lower, with aromatase inhibitors [36]. As with chemotherapy, the risk of treatment with hormonal agents needs to be weighed against the benefits of treatment. Patients may have several pre-existing risks for developing clots, such as smoking, hypertension, irritable bowel syndrome, obesity, and/or personal or family history of clotting [37]. With multiple clotting risks, treatments other than hormones may be prudent.

Tests showing cardiac dysfunction may include EKG changes, decreased LVEF or anatomic disturbances on ECHO or MUGA, cardiomegaly (enlarged heart) on chest radiography, thromboembolism on Doppler imaging, hypokinesis of myocardium on stress imaging, and stenosed arteries with catheterization [36]. Laboratory findings may include abnormalities in arterial blood gases, complete blood cell counts, chemistry panels, troponins, brain natriuretic peptide, C-reactive protein, D-dimer, and homocysteine [36–38].

Strategies for treatment and improvements in technology have diminished the long-term effects of CIC. Improved radiation therapy techniques that shield the heart, frequent cardiac screening, appropriate and prompt drug cessation or dose reductions, and intervention with cardioprotective medications help decrease CIC [39]. Dexrazoxane (Zinecard), a cardioprotectant chelating agent when infused with doxorubicin given by IVP, has been shown to decrease the development of CHF by 19% [40]. Dexrazoxane is not recommended for use at the beginning of anthracycline therapy because of the possibility that it might reduce the anticancer effects of the anthracycline [6].

Stratification of risk factors is important in predicting the development of CIC when treatment using cardiotoxic chemotherapeutic and biologic agents is necessary. In patients who had elevated serum troponin I levels, 80% developed a 15% reduction in left ventricular dysfunction [23]. Cardinale and colleagues [41] randomly assigned 114 patients who had elevated troponin levels after treatment with high-dose chemotherapy (including anthracyclines) to receive either prophylactic enalapril, an angiotensin-converting enzyme (ace) inhibitor, or placebo for 1 year. The enalapril group had no left ventricular dysfunction but 43% of the placebo group developed a decrease in LV function of 10% or more [41]. Animal studies of the prophylactic use of erythropoietin and thrombopoietin to prevent or decrease the incidence of CIC development are ongoing [42,43].

Once CIC occurs, treatment is directed at addressing specific symptom manifestations. The mainstays of treatment for left ventricular dysfunction, CHF, and cardiomyopathy are angiotensin-converting enzyme inhibitors, beta-blockers, and diuretics [6]. If venous thromboembolism occurs, treatment options include thrombolytic infusion, anticoagulation, use of compression stockings, and elevation of the affected extremity (personal communication, A. Kommareddy, 2007).

Case study

A 47-year-old married white woman was diagnosed with stage IIIA right breast cancer in September 2005. Her tumor was estrogen-receptor (ER) and progesterone-receptor (PR) negative and HER2-receptor positive. Mild hypertension before diagnosis had been controlled with the angiotensin-converting enzyme inhibitor enalapril (Vasotec). Her baseline ejection fraction measured by ECHO was 55%. She had a right mastectomy followed by immediate reconstruction. Treatment with doxorubicin was started by continuous infusion to a total dose of 240 mg/m^2 and cyclophosphamide for four cycles. This regimen was followed by right chest radiation and then four cycles of paclitaxel with trastuzumab. The treatment was followed with maintenance trastuzumab beginning in May 2006.

The patient presented to the emergency department with new-onset dyspnea and viral pneumonia in March 2007. The ECHO showed an ejection fraction of 15% to 20%. Possible causes for the cardiomyopathy included doxorubicin treatment, trastuzumab treatment, viral pneumonia, and controlled hypertension. Given the low dose of doxorubicin and its administration by continuous infusion, doxorubicin was unlikely to be the cause of the CIC. Trastuzumab CIC was a possibility, but intercurrent infection or other conditions might have caused this cardiomyopathy. Cardiology treated and stabilized the patient with diuretics and beta-blockers. She was released on a regimen of carvedilol (Coreg) and aspirin. Over 8 months her ejection fraction improved to baseline.

When the patient complained of right upper quadrant pain in October 2007, she was diagnosed as having liver and right pelvic metastases. Further treatment for cancer was required. With her history of compromised cardiac function, she was treated with gemcitabine and albumin-bound paclitaxel, drugs with relatively low risk for CIC [19,20]. With her cancer now controlled, and at the patient's request, consideration is being given to rechallenging her with trastuzumab for maintenance treatment with careful cardiac monitoring and collaboration with her treating cardiologist. Although her disease is considered incurable, control of disease progression may enhance this patient's quality of life. Her survival depends on treatment sustaining long-term control of her ER-negative, PR-negative, and *HER2*-positive disease.

As with many chronic illnesses requiring complex treatment and rehabilitation, patients often are unable to work. The patient in the case study missed several weeks of work because of her illness, surgery, recovery, treatment, and complications, creating difficult socioeconomic issues affecting both the patient and her family. She ultimately lost her employment because of absenteeism exceeding that allowed by the Family Medical Leave Act. She continues to be insured through her husband's employment but does not have secondary coverage. She probably will be unlikely able to obtain insurance on her own in the future. Her disease has affected all facets of her and her family's life, physically, emotionally and financially.

References

[1] American Cancer Society. Cancer statistics 2007. Available at: http://www.cancer.org/docroot/PRO/content/PRO_1_1_Cancer_Statistics_2007_Presentation.asp. Accessed December 20, 2007.

[2] About breast cancer: statistics, causes, symptoms, surgery options. Available at: http://www.breastcancer.org. Accessed December 2007.

[3] Facts for life breast cancer in men. Susan G. Komen for the Cure Web site. Available at: http://cms.

komen.org/Komen/AboutBreastCancer/Resources. Updated 2007. Accessed December 2007.

[4] Surveillance Epidemiology and End Results Program. Available at: http://seer.cancer.gov. Accessed December 2007.

[5] Multiple hit hypothesis: how breast cancer treatment affects heart disease in women. Her2 Support Group Forum Web site. Available at: http://www.her2support.org. Accessed December 2007.

[6] Yeh ETH, Tong AT, Lenihan DJ, et al. Cardiovascular complications of cancer therapy: diagnosis, pathogenesis, and management. Circulation 2004; 109(25):3122–31.

[7] O'Toole M. Miller-Keane encyclopedia and dictionary of medicine, nursing, and allied health. 5th edition. Philadelphia: W.B.Saunders Company; 1992.

[8] Adriamycin [package insert]. Bedford (OH): Ben Venue Laboratories, Inc. and Bedford Laboratories; 2006.

[9] Kozier B, Erb G, Olivieri R. Fundamentals of nursing concepts process and practice. 4th edition. Redwood City (CA): Benjamin/Cummings Publishing Co, Inc.; 1991. p. 408–11.

[10] Beers MH, Berkow R. The Merck manual. 17th edition. Whitehouse (NJ): Merck Research Laboratories; 1999.

[11] Singhal H. Breast cancer evaluation. Emedicine Web site. Available at: http://www.emedicine.com/med/topic3287.htm. Accessed January 2008.

[12] American Cancer Society. How is breast cancer staged? Available at: http://wwwcancer.org. Updated September 13, 2007. Accessed December 2007.

[13] National Comprehensive Cancer Network. Practice guidelines in oncology—v.1.2008. Breast cancer. ST-1-3. National Comprehensive Cancer Network (NCCN) Web site. Available at: http://www.nccn.org/professionals/physician_gls/PDF/breast.pdf. Accessed December 2007.

[14] Jones LW, Haykowsky M, Pituskin EN, et al. Cardiovascular reserve and risk profile of postmenopausal women after chemoendocrine therapy for hormone receptor-positive operable breast cancer. Oncologist 2007;12(10):1156–64. Available at: http://theoncologist.alphamedpress.org/cgi/content/abstract/12/10/1156. Accessed January 2008.

[15] Oparil S. The importance of identifying and reducing cardiovascular risk factors in women. Available at: http://www.medscape.com/viewarticle/448971_5. Accessed January 2008.

[16] National Institutes of Health. Estimating coronary heart disease (CHD) risk using Framingham Heart Study prediction score sheets. Available at: http://www.nhlbi.nih.gov/about/framingham/riskabs.htm. Accessed January 2008.

[17] Calculating heart and stroke risk for women. Reynolds Risk Score Web site. Available at: http://www.reynoldsriskscore.org/. Accessed January 2008.

[18] Mays T. Oncology Preparatory Review Course Handbook. The American College of Clinical Pharmacy and the American Society of Health-System Pharmacists; 2007.

[19] Gemzar [package insert]. Indianapolis (IN): Eli Lilly and Company; 2006.

[20] Abraxane [package insert]. Los Angeles (CA): Abraxis Oncology, Division of Abraxis BioScience, Inc.; 2007.

[21] Doxil [package insert]. Bedford (OH): Ben Venue Laboratories, Inc.; 2006.

[22] Herceptin [package insert]. South San Francisco (CA): Genentech, Inc.; 2006.

[23] Granger CB. Prediction and prevention of chemotherapy-induced cardiomyopathy: can it be done? Circulation 2006;114(23):2432–3.

[24] National Comprehensive Cancer Network. Practice guidelines in oncology—v.1.2008. Invasive breast cancer. BINV-I, BINV-J 1-5, BINV–M 1-6. Available at: http://www.nccn.org/professionals/physi cian_gls/PDF/breast.pdf. Updated January 2008. Accessed January 1, 2008.

[25] Simbre II VC, Adams J, Deshpande SS, et al. Cardiomyopathy caused by antineoplastic therapies. Curr Treat Options Cardiovasc Med 2001;3:493–505. Available at: http://www.treatment-options.com. Accessed January 2008.

[26] US Food and Drug Administration. Guidance for industry. Available at: http://www.fda.gov/cber/ gdlns/boxwarlb.htm. Updated January 20, 2006. Accessed December 28, 2007.

[27] Hortobaygi GN, Frye D, Buzdar AU, et al. Decreased cardiac toxicity of doxorubicin administered by continuous intravenous infusion in combination chemotherapy for metastatic breast carcinoma. Cancer 1989;63(1):37–45.

[28] National Cancer Institute. Dictionary of cancer terms. Available at: http://www.cancer/gov/Tem plates/db_alpha.aspx?expand=M. Accessed January 1, 2008.

[29] The genes of cancer: oncogenes. HER-2/neu. Emory University Web site. Available at: http://www.cancerquest. org/index.cfm?page=325. Accessed January 2008.

[30] Hortobaygi GN. Trastuzumab in the treatment of breast cancer. N Engl J Med 2005;353(16): 1734–6.

[31] Smith M. SABCS: one-third of HER2-positive breast tumors metastasize to brain. MedPage Today Web site. Available at: http://www.medpagetoday. com/MeetingCoverage/SABCSMeeting/tb/7721. Accessed January 2008.

[32] Burstein HJ. The distinctive nature of HER2-positive breast cancers. N Engl J Med 2005; 353(16):1652–4.

[33] Romond E. Joint analysis of NSABP-B-31 and NCCTG –N9831. American Society of Clinical Oncology (ASCO) Web site. Available at: http:// media.asco.org/player/default.aspx?LectureID=5817& conferenceFolder=VM2005&SessionFolder=ss11& slideonlu=yes&TrackIBN929&LectureTitle. Accessed December 10, 2007.

[34] Avastin [package insert]. South San Francisco (CA): Genentech, Inc.; 2006.

[35] Nolvadex [package insert]. Wilminton (DE): Astra Zeneca Pharmaceuticals; 2002.

[36] Arimidex [package insert]. Wilmington (DE): Astra Zeneca Pharmaceuticals; 2006.

[37] Heit JA. Prevention of deep venous thrombosis. In: Dalsing MC, editor. The vein handbook: a layman's versions of venous disorders. American Venous Forum Web site. Available at: http://www.venous-info. com/handbook/hbk10a.html. Accessed December 30, 2007.

[38] Camp-Sorrell D. Cardiorespiratory effects in cancer survivors: cardiac and pulmonary toxicities may occur as late or long-term sequelae of cancer treatment. Am J Nursing 2006;106(Suppl 3):55–9.

[39] Zinecard [package insert]. Kalamazoo (MI): Pharmacia and Upjohn; 1998.

[40] Cardinale D, Sandri M, Colombo A, et al. Prognostic value of troponin I in cardiac risk stratification of cancer patients undergoing high-dose chemotherapy. Circulation 2004;109(22):2749–54.

[41] Cardinale D, Colombo A, Sandri M, et al. Prevention of high-dose chemotherapy-induced cardiotoxicity in high-risk patients by angiotensin-converting enzyme inhibition. Circulation 2006; 114(23):2474–81.

[42] Li l, Takemura G, Li Y, et al. Preventative effect of erythropoietin on cardiac dysfunction in doxorubicin-induced cardiomyopathy. Circulation 2006; 113(4):535–43.

[43] Li K, Sung R, Huang W, et al. Thrombopoietin protects against in vitro and in vivo cardiotoxicity induced by doxorubicin. Circulation 2006;113(18): 2211–20.

CRITICAL CARE
NURSING CLINICS
OF NORTH AMERICA

Crit Care Nurs Clin N Am 20 (2008) 351–357

Why Women Need to Sweat: The Benefits of Cardiac Rehabilitation

Lori Barron, BSN, RN, BC[a],*,
Lynn Smith Schnautz, RN, MSN, CCRN, CCNS, NP-C[b,c]

[a]Cardiac Rehabilitation, Deaconess Hospital, 415 West Columbia Street, Evansville, IN 47710, USA
[b]Deaconess Hospital, 600 Mary Street, Evansville, IN 47747, USA
[c]Integrity Family Physicians, 6221 East Physicians Court, Evansville, IN 47715, USA

The updated guidelines from the American Heart Association declare that most women in the United States are at risk for cardiovascular disease (CVD), a situation that calls for a long-term approach to preventing and treating the condition. CVD is the leading cause of death of women and kills more women than men in the United States yearly [1].

In 1995, the Agency for Health Care Policy and Research funded a broad scientific review of outcomes associated with cardiac rehabilitation (CR) programs. This review showed that people who participated in CR programs have a 20% to 25% decrease in death from heart disease (American Association of Cardiovascular and Pulmonary Rehabilitation [AACVPR]) [2]. Even though there is strong evidence supporting CR programs, they are underutilized. Only 20% to 30% of patients who are appropriate candidates for CR are referred to these programs, and some studies indicate that as few as 10% to 20% participate [3].

Women typically are about 10 years older than men when they initially exhibit symptoms of CVD. Symptom presentation often is different in women than in men. Crushing chest pain is less common, and many women have atypical symptoms such as a gastrointestinal or flulike presentation [2]. According to Patricia Davidson, Chief Researcher and Associate Professor from the University of Western Sydney, women are not encouraged as strongly as men to participate

in CR programs after they are discharged from the hospital. Women also are more inclined to subordinate their health needs to the needs of their partner, children, work, and other commitments [4]. When a patient is experiencing a life-threatening event, that is the ideal time to provide education regarding lifestyle changes that directly affect heart-healthy living. For critical care health care providers, who act as patient advocates, this is an opportune time to provide education to patients who have CVD about the benefits or CR.

History of cardiac rehabilitation

In the 1930s, patients who had a myocardial infarction were advised to observe 6 weeks of bed rest. Chair therapy was introduced in the 1940s. By the early 1950s, 3 to 5 minutes of daily walking was advocated, beginning 4 weeks after the event. Clinicians gradually began to recognize that early ambulation avoided many of the complications of bed rest, including pulmonary embolism. Concerns about the safety of unsupervised exercise remained strong and led to the development of structured physician-supervised rehabilitation programs that included EKG monitoring.

In the 1950s, Hellerstein established one of the first CR programs for patients recovering from acute cardiac events. He advocated a multidisciplinary approach to the rehabilitation program [5].

What is cardiac rehabilitation?

CR is much more than simply exercise. It is a medically based program in which patients are

* Corresponding author.
E-mail address: lori_barron@deaconess.com
(L. Barron).

0899-5885/08/$ - see front matter © 2008 Elsevier Inc. All rights reserved.
doi:10.1016/j.ccell.2008.03.005

provided with a medical evaluation, a prescribed exercise regimen, and education and counseling regarding CVD. Individuals who do not have heart disease also may participate in a CR program to be educated regarding heart disease prevention and maintenance of a heart healthy lifestyle.

CR provides both comprehensive and individualized plans of care. Short-term goals include sufficient reconditioning to allow resumption of customary activities, limiting the physiologic and psychologic effects of heart disease, decreasing the risk of sudden cardiac arrest or reinfarction, and controlling the symptoms of cardiac disease. Long-term goals include identification and treatment of risk factors, stabilizing or even reversing the atherosclerotic process, and enhancing the psychologic status of the patients [5].

Patient selection

Entry into CR requires a physician's order, but anyone may discuss CR with the patient and family. Initial discussion of a CR program should begin in the hospital. The bedside nurse is one of the key players in recommending and explaining the importance and benefits of CR. Most commercial insurance companies, along with Medicare and Medicaid, provide some reimbursement for early outpatient CR with approved diagnoses. Diagnoses that typically are covered include percutaneous coronary angioplasty, myocardial infarction, angina, coronary artery bypass surgery, and valvular heart surgery and heart transplantation. Candidacy for entry into the program also may include stable heart failure, peripheral arterial disease with claudication, and/or other forms of CVD [3].

Many patients state that CR was not discussed with them in the hospital and that they first heard about the program when a member of the CR team telephoned them after discharge. Also, many patients participate because of word-of-mouth reports from other patients who have benefited from CR.

Health care providers need to know where CR facilities are located and whom a patient should contact to enroll in a program. Several CR programs offer a day of observation so health care providers can witness first hand the benefits of an effective program.

Contraindications

Some disease states contraindicate patients' participation in a CR program. These conditions include unstable ischemia, heart failure that is not compensated, uncontrolled arrhythmias, severe and symptomatic aortic stenosis, hypertrophic obstructive cardiomyopathy, severe pulmonary hypertension, and other conditions that could be aggravated by exercise (ie, resting systolic blood pressure $\geq$ 200 mm Hg or resting diastolic blood pressure $\geq$ 110 mm Hg), active or suspected myocarditis or pericarditis, suspected or known dissecting aneurysm, thrombophlebitis, or recent systemic or pulmonary embolism [2].

Phases of cardiac rehabilitation

Cardiac rehabilitation and secondary prevention programs are a vital part of the continuum of care. Inpatient CR begins in the hospital when a patient is recovering from a cardiovascular event. Patients are educated about the signs and symptoms of heart disease, when to seek medical attention, how to follow medication instructions, and how to increase their exercise progressively beginning with walking in the halls. Early outpatient CR (commonly known as "phase II CR") starts within 1 to 2 weeks after the cardiovascular event, with emphasis on risk-factor education, counseling, and exercise. It usually lasts 4 to 12 weeks and usually is provided at an outpatient CR facility. Maintenance and follow-up (commonly known as "phase III CR") often begins 2 to 3 months after the event. These classes may be held at various locations, such as the hospital, a community exercise facility, a YMCA, a college gymnasium, and/or a commercial health center. Compliance can be monitored by onsite checkups, telephone, e-mail, and/or mailed surveys [2].

Getting started

Once an order is obtained for outpatient CR, an initial visit is scheduled. A low-level treadmill test or 6-minute walk test is given to assess the patient's energy level and target heart rate while exercising. The past medical history is obtained along with information about risk factors to help the team set up the individualized program to fit the patient's needs. Many patients who have heart disease have comorbidities such as diabetes, heart failure, chronic obstructive pulmonary disease, asthma, cardiomyopathy, arthritis, back problems, knee or hip replacements, chronic fatigue syndrome, and/or depression. All these conditions must be considered in designing the patient's exercise program.

To someone who has had a cardiovascular event, life can seem overwhelming. The beauty of CR is that it allows nurses and exercise specialists to give patients information a little at a time to help alleviate their fears. Risk factors are discussed with the patient, and then goals with a plan of action are determined. Risk factors for heart disease that should be discussed with the patient include smoking history, nutrition, exercise patterns, weight management, diabetes, hypertension, and stress management. Developing a good health habit usually takes about 3 months, so it is extremely important for the patient to start a CR program as quickly as possible and to participate for the full duration of the program.

Patients are instructed to exercise in CR classes up to three times a week and are encouraged to exercise on their own on the days when they do not attend CR classes. The duration and intensity varies from patient to patient. Some patients may be able to exercise only 5 minutes or less, but others may begin by exercising for 15 or 20 minutes without a rest period. Patients need to allow 30 to 60 minutes for each session, which includes warm-up and cool-down periods of at least 5 to 10 minutes each. Blood pressure, heart rate, perceived exertion scale, and discomfort are factored into the plan.

Cardiac rehabilitation classes

Education to prevent further cardiovascular events and slow the progression of heart disease is vital. Education is presented in a variety of ways through formalized classes that meet daily or weekly or on a need-to-know basis in one-on-one sessions. Topics may vary, but core classes typically include

- Understanding CVD
- Medication guidelines
- Coping with stress
- Diabetes and exercise
- Facts about hypertension
- Heart-healthy eating
- Exercise
- Smoking

Many topics are covered in CR education, but it is especially important that patients learn about CVD. Education about CVD may include information on the anatomy of the heart, the coronary arteries, and the heart's electrical system. Symptoms of angina, myocardial infarction, and stroke are discussed, along with instructions about what to do if these symptoms occur. Procedures used to treat coronary artery disease such as coronary angioplasty, stenting, coronary artery bypass grafting, pacemakers, and implantable cardiac defibrillators are reviewed. Actual examples of stents, pacemakers, and implantable defibrillators are shown to the patients.

A medication review emphasizes the importance of taking medicines properly as they have been prescribed. Education is provided regarding when, why, and how to take the medications; the importance of carrying an updated medication list, and encouraging the use of one pharmacy to decrease the risk of medication errors. Patients often have many questions regarding medications, and this education is an important part of the continued success of follow-up care.

Exercise has been shown to decrease symptoms of depression, and learning to cope with stress is another important topic. The inability to cope with excessive stress can affect physical and mental well being. As Hamer [6] stated, "Chronic stressors such as low socioeconomic status, work stress, marital stress, caregiver strain, low social support and emotional factors linked with stress such as depression, are associated with an increased risk of CVD development." The guidelines of the AACVPR [2] warn that "Female coronary patients who have fewer psychosocial supports, are more likely to be depressed, and are more likely to live alone than male patients. The presence of depression predicts not only a worsened cardiac prognosis for those afflicted, but poorer physical functioning and quality of life." Being aware of some of the symptoms of stress, such as tight neck and shoulder muscles, fatigue, irritability, and impatience, is the first step in controlling stress. Stress-reducing strategies that are taught may include relaxation, exercising, talking to a friend, confronting the situation, prioritizing responsibilities, doing something for oneself, and seeking professional help if nothing seems to work. Additional ways of coping with stress may include adjusting attitudes and goals, rehearsing stressful situations mentally, avoiding stressful situations, managing time, organizing work, and setting priorities. Getting enough rest is also of great importance.

General diabetes management and exercise is reviewed, because "CVD is the most common complication of diabetes in women, and diabetes is the only condition that causes women to have rates of CVD similar to those of men" [7]. Some of the guidelines that are discussed with patients are to carry foods that provide quick energy while exercising, to wear cotton socks and good supportive shoes, and to check feet for cuts, blisters, and reddened areas before and after exercise. It also is important to eat regular meals at about the same time each day. The combination of weight loss and increased activity can lower blood sugar, so it is extremely important to check blood glucose levels before and after exercise. Insulin dosages may have to be decreased, and feedback to the physician is essential.

Interaction with the CR staff in the training environment may enhance the patient's social support, which in turn may play an important role in improving mood and is likely to increase the antihypertensive effects of exercise training [8] (Fig. 1). Blood pressure classifications are discussed, and ways to control hypertension are provided (Table 1). By maintaining a healthy weight, avoiding excessive alcohol use, not smoking, exercising regularly, reducing stress, controlling diabetes, cutting down on salty foods, and eating more fresh fruits and vegetables, patients are able to reach their goals.

Heart-healthy eating is a major topic that is covered. General information is discussed, such as choosing foods that are low in fat, cholesterol, and sodium and eating fresh fruits and vegetables, whole-grain breads and pastas, low-fat dairy products, and lean cuts of meat, fish, and poultry. Basic information about saturated, polyunsaturated, and monounsaturated fats is reviewed. Patients are taught to read labels for fat, cholesterol, and sodium content. Visual aids such as the food guide pyramid and using the palm of the hand as a measure for portion control are helpful resources. The area of the palm is equivalent to a serving of 3 ounces of cooked meat; the size of the fist is equivalent to 1 cup (ie, two servings) of pasta or oatmeal; a thumb tip is equivalent to 1 teaspoon of margarine, a thumb is equivalent to 1 ounce of cheese, and a handful of snack foods such as peanuts is approximately 1 ounce.

Healthier ways of cooking food, such as roasting, baking, poaching, grilling, broiling, sautéing, or steaming, are discussed also. Substitutions are suggested that make recipes healthier (eg, using egg whites in place of yolks, substituting apple sauce for oil when baking, using herbs and spices in place of salt to add flavor to food, and using low-fat cottage cheese plus low-fat or nonfat yogurt in place of sour cream). Learning to keep a record of what the patient has eaten reinforces the making of good

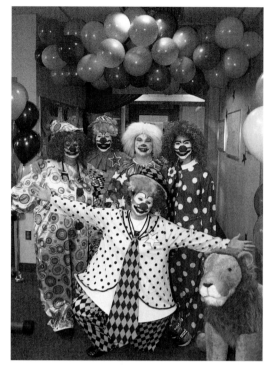

Fig. 1. Cardiac rehabilitation celebrates life: Susie Kirsch, Lori Griffin, Lori Barron, Ginny Waters, and Staci Hodges. At Deaconess Hospital CR, the nursing staff and exercise specialists remind themselves daily that this is a time of uncertainty in the lives of their patients. Each October the CR staff transforms the facility into a lighthearted, fun-loving place where, for just 1 day, the patients do not need to think about CVD. (Photograph *courtesy of* Dave Waller, Production Photographer, Team Leader, A-V Department, Deaconess Hospital, Evansville, Indiana.)

food choices and allows a person to evaluate his or her eating habits honestly. A dietician is available for consultation if desired.

Physical inactivity is a risk factor for developing coronary artery disease. When starting CR, patients' knowledge and levels of physical activity vary greatly. Some patients have been active all their lives; others have not. According to the AACVPR, "Women are less fit at entry to CR than men, even when the age difference is not significant" [2]. It is important for patients to start "slow and low" but just start moving! Activity does wonderful things for the body: lowering blood glucose levels and blood pressure, helping with weight loss, increasing the body's use of and sensitivity to insulin, improving strength and physical-working capacity, sharpening the

Table 1
Classification and management of blood pressure for adults aged 18 years or older

Parameter				Management		
				Lifestyle modification	Initial drug therapy	
Blood pressure classification	Systolic blood pressure (mm Hg[a])		Diastolic blood pressure (mm Hg[a])		Without compelling indication	With compelling indications
Normal	< 120	and	< 80	Encourage		
Prehypertension	120–139	or	80–89	Yes	No antihypertensive drug indicated	Drug(s) for the compelling indications[b]
Stage 1 hypertension	140–159	or	90–99	Yes	Thiazide-type diuretics for most; may consider ACE inhibitor, ARB, BB, CCB, or combination	Drug(s) for the compelling indications. Other antihypertensive drugs (diuretic, ACE inhibitor, ARB, BB, CCB) as needed.
Stage 2 hypertension	≥ 160	or	≥ 100	Yes	Two-drug combination for most (usually thiazide-type diuretic and ACE inhibitor or ARB or BB or CCB)[c]	Drug(s) for the compelling indications. Other antihypertensive drugs (diuretics, ACE inhibitor, ARB, BB) needed.

Abbreviations: ACE, angiotensin-converting enzyme; ARB, angiotensin-receptor blocker; BB, beta-blocker; CCB, calcium-channel blocker; DBP, diastolic blood pressure; SBP, systolic blood pressure.

[a] Treatment determined by highest category.

[b] Treat patients who have chronic kidney disease or diabetes to blood pressure goal of < 130/80 mm Hg.

[c] Initial combined therapy should be used cautiously in patients at risk for orthostatic hypotension.

Data from National Cholesterol Education Program (NCEP). Executive summary of the third report of the Expert Panel on Detection, Evaluation and Treatment of High Blood Cholesterol in Adults (Adult Treatment Panel III). JAMA 2003;289(19):2560–72.

mind, and toning the body. Exercise helps increase high-density lipoprotein levels and reduces triglyceride levels and stress. Proper warm-up and cool-down on the equipment are reviewed, along with weight guidelines and restrictions. Guidelines for exercising in hot and cold weather are provided also. At times, it is hard for patients to stay motivated; developing a buddy system may keep a patient on track. CR offers a support system and accountability. The patients always know if a classmate is absent from CR and may follow up with a contact to make sure the patient is okay.

Smoking cessation is discussed with the patient and/or family if desired. General facts about smoking and about second-hand smoking are discussed. For patients who are ready to quit, information and follow-up are given regarding formalized smoking cessation classes. For others tips for quitting, cues, alternatives, constant praise, and follow-up are provided. When a patient is not ready to quit, discussion and education center on informing the patient about the help that is available and about letting the nursing staff know when the patient is ready to stop smoking. The subject of smoking is reviewed periodically during the patient's CR visits to see if the patient is ready to quit.

Outcomes

An effective CR program has many documented benefits. Physical benefits include improved exercise tolerance and the reduction of risk factors that include the lowering of lipid levels, blood pressure, body weight, and blood glucose level. Patients gain better control of their symptoms. Psychologic improvements include reduction in stress, anxiety, and depression; enhanced social adjustment and functioning; and increased rate of return to work. Reductions in mortality rate also have been well documented in the literature [5].

Julie's red dress

Julie is a 30-year-old white woman who has a history of tetralogy of Fallott, an anomaly of the heart consisting of pulmonary stenosis, interventricular septal defect, dextroposed aorta that receives blood from both ventricles, and hypertrophy of the right ventricle [9] (Fig. 2). At 8 months of age, Julie underwent unsuccessful open-heart surgery. A second attempt at repair was made at 18 months of age and again was unsuccessful. One day later, a successful repair was achieved. Julie did well until age 23 years, when she developed heart failure. She was at work one evening and she told her co-workers that she

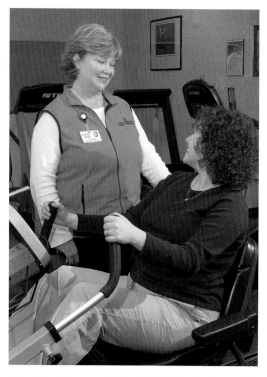

Fig. 2. Lori Barron, RN, and Julie Stucki, former CR patient and current exercise specialist. (Photograph *courtesy of* Dave Waller, Production Photographer, Team Leader, A-V Department, Deaconess Hospital, Evansville, Indiana.)

"didn't feel right." She was working in a hospital, so her co-workers attached her to a heart monitor that revealed sinus tachycardia with a heart rate of 170 beats/minute, and her pulse oximetry was in the 80s. She was sent to her family doctor, who sent her to Riley Hospital in Indianapolis the next day. An adjustment was made to her medications, and she discontinued birth-control pills. In February 2007, she saw her doctor for a check-up at the request of her mother who recently had read an article regarding children who had undergone surgery for tetralogy of Fallot repairs as youngsters. Julie had gained 20 pounds and was taking 2-hour naps daily. She stated that taking naps had been her routine for so long that she had not realized that she was in heart failure, because she had learned to compensate. In May 2007, at the age of 28 years, she had a pulmonary valve replacement. Julie has worked in health care since the age of 18 years, and a friend suggested that she attend a CR program. According to Julie, the CR program had many benefits. She stated that CR was a great social event and support group. The staff was very knowledgeable, and she learned many heart-healthy lifestyle modifications in the classes. The nutrition class was exceptional, and she learned a great deal about reading food labels. "Attending CR makes you get up and go. You are pretty sore but if you move you feel so much better." She reports that one of the greatest advantages of attending CR was meeting three wonderful friends. She spent her twenty-ninth birthday at CR, and one of the women brought her a birthday mug. She said, "Whether you are 29 or 79, you share something in common." The three close friends she made in CR continue their friendship today and have lunch together once a month. Julie now works in CR as an exercise specialist. Julie stated that one thing that made a profound impression on her was a statement she heard when she was in high school: "Never tell a patient you know what they are going through." She said she now knows she can tell the CR patients that she knows first hand what they are experiencing, and she shares a special bond with them.

Summary

CR is an essential component in the recovery of patients from cardiovascular disease. CR involves exercise training, education, counseling regarding lifestyle modification, and behavior interventions. The goals of CR are to improve both the physiologic and psychosocial condition of the patient. Physical benefits include improvement of exercise capacity and reduction of risk factors including decreased smoking and the lowering of lipid levels, weight, blood pressure, and blood glucose level. Psychologic improvements include reduction in stress, anxiety, and depression. Knowing the benefits of an effective CR program will help critical care nurses and physicians promote and refer patients who have CVD into this life-changing, heart-healthy program.

Acknowledgment

The authors thank Dr. Jerry Becker, medical director, and the nurses and exercise specialists at Deaconess Hospital Outpatient Cardiac Rehabilitation Department for assisting and supporting in this endeavor.

References

[1] Traynor K. Heart disease prevention recommendations revised for women. Am J Health Syst Pharm 2007;64(7):680.

[2] American Association of Cardiovascular and Pulmonary Rehabilitation. Guidelines for the cardiac rehabilitation and secondary prevention programs. 4th edition. Champaign (IL): Human Kinetics; 2004. p. 72, 140–41.

[3] Leon AS, Franklin BA, Costa F, et al. Cardiac rehabilitation and secondary prevention of coronary heart disease. Circulation 2005;111:369–76.

[4] Focus. Neurological, rehabilitation, education. Cardiac rehab program gets women going again. (June 2005). Australian Nursing Journal. Available at: http://webebscohost.com.lib-proxy.usi.edu/ehost/delivery?vid+10&;hid+108&sid=c35c02. Accessed September 25, 2007.

[5] Singh VN, Schocken DD, Williams K, et al. Cardiac rehabilitation. March 28, 2006. Available at: http://www.emedicine.com/pmr/topic180.htm. Accessed January 14, 2008 1–16.

[6] Hamer M. Exercise and psychobiological processes. Sports Med 2006;36(10):829–38.

[7] Rosenfield AG. State of the heart: building science to improve women's cardiovascular health. Am J Crit Care 2006;15:556–66.

[8] Hamer M. The anti-hypertensive effects of exercise. Sports Med 2006;36(2):109–16.

[9] Davis FA. Taber's cyclopedic medical dictitionary. 18th edition. Philadelphia: FA Davis Company; 1993. p. 1931.

ELSEVIER
SAUNDERS

Crit Care Nurs Clin N Am 20 (2008) 359–364

CRITICAL CARE
NURSING CLINICS
OF NORTH AMERICA

Index

Note: Page numbers of article titles are in **boldface** type.

0899-5885/08/$ - see front matter © 2008 Elsevier Inc. All rights reserved.
doi:10.1016/S0899-5885(08)00045-2

ccnursing.theclinics.com

Moving?

Make sure your subscription moves with you!

To notify us of your new address, find your **Clinics Account Number** (located on your mailing label above your name), and contact customer service at:

E-mail: elspcs@elsevier.com

800-654-2452 (subscribers in the U.S. & Canada)
1-407-563-6020 (subscribers outside of the U.S. & Canada)

Fax number: 407-363-9661

Elsevier Periodicals Customer Service
6277 Sea Harbor Drive
Orlando, FL 32887-4800

*To ensure uninterrupted delivery of your subscription, please notify us at least 4 weeks in advance of move.